Praise for *But You* Look *Fine*

"Amy Kurtz exposes a common occurrence that until now has gone unnamed and undiscussed by doctors and patients alike. Not only does she reveal this roadblock to wellness, but she also offers solutions, ones that we can all apply to our lives, whether chronically ill, newly diagnosed, or labeled 'cured.' This is a paradigm-shifting book and a must-read."

—MARK HYMAN, MD, #1 *NEW YORK TIMES* BESTSELLING AUTHOR AND HOST OF *THE DR. HYMAN SHOW*

"If you or a loved one suffer from invisible chronic illness, *But You* Look *Fine* is essential reading. Through its pages, Amy Kurtz presents a structured program that will immeasurably enhance your journey toward healing."

—LEO GALLAND, MD, BESTSELLING AUTHOR AND BOARD-CERTIFIED INTERNIST SPECIALIZING IN THE TREATMENT OF PATIENTS WITH CHRONIC COMPLEX ILLNESS

"*But You* Look *Fine* offers clarity, compassion and a rare blend of scientific rigor and heartfelt guidance. It's an empowering guide that gifts readers the tools needed to move forward with clarity and purpose in their quest for regaining stewardship over their health destiny."

—DAVID PERLMUTTER, MD, FACN, #1 *NEW YORK TIMES* BESTSELLING AUTHOR OF *GRAIN BRAIN* AND *BRAIN DEFENDERS*

"Amy Kurtz shares something in this book that is rarely talked about from the patient's perspective. It is wise, insightful, fearless, and provides you tools, not just reasons. In a sea of books about well-being, if you've struggled with illness, grab this one first."

—SHELLEY KOLTON, MD

"Amy Kurtz's vulnerable account is a testament to the enduring human spirit. *But You* Look *Fine* isn't just about surviving chronic illness; it's about thriving in its aftermath. It's a wellspring of courage, resilience, and the unwavering belief that even after hitting bottom, you can rise, stronger, wiser, and more resilient."

—KRIS CARR, *NEW YORK TIMES* BESTSELLING AUTHOR, WELLNESS ACTIVIST, AND CANCER THRIVER

"A tapestry woven of emergent resilience, commitment, and trust, *But You* Look *Fine* is a must for anyone who's ever been lost in the labyrinth of illness. Amy Kurtz is the knowing voice of a good friend offering guidance with humility, presence, and clarity."

—ELENA BROWER, BESTSELLING AUTHOR OF *HOLD NOTHING* AND *PRACTICE YOU*

"With introspection yet fierce spirit, Amy Kurtz navigates the uncharted territory of what whole healing really means. This book is an essential read for anyone who has stared into the abyss of illness and emerged forever changed. I am so grateful she is bringing this tremendously important perspective of healing out of the shadows and into the light."

—JOEL EVANS, MD, FORMER CHIEF OF MEDICAL AFFAIRS, THE INSTITUTE FOR FUNCTIONAL MEDICINE

"If chronic illness feels like being at war with oneself, Amy Kurtz offers an answer. Her book, *But You* Look *Fine*, is the key for those struggling to find their way back to health. It's a testament to the power of vulnerability, a call to arms for those fighting unseen battles. This book is a trailblazing read for anyone yearning to break the shackles of illness and move into a future filled with possibility."

—DR. GABRIELLE LYON, DO, *NEW YORK TIMES* BESTSELLING AUTHOR OF *FOREVER STRONG*

"Amy's book is ultimately one about righteous sight. She casts light on the millions of lived chronic patient experiences longing for a rewrite, and with her trademark warmth and championship, guides those waiting to leave the shadows of illness. With the intimacy and emboldening of a coaching session and from the authenticity of a fellow warrior, she transforms our inner lens so that it can correct our external world's vision. Prepare for crystal-clear, 20/20 patient empowerment."

—SARA HIRSH BORDO, AWARD-WINNING FILMMAKER AND AUTHOR OF *AUTOIMMUNITY AND THE GOOD GIRLS*

"Recognizing the mental, physical, and emotional toll that western healing can take on patients, Amy Kurtz creates a workable roadmap to holistic health in *But You* Look *Fine*. With kindness, compassion, and humor Kurtz guides readers through life after chronic illness, through what can be an otherwise bewildering and uncharted land."

—SHARON SALZBERG, MEDITATION PIONEER, WORLD-RENOWNED TEACHER, AND *NEW YORK TIMES* BESTSELLING AUTHOR

"*But You* Look *Fine* gives voice to a painful dimension of chronic illness that is rarely acknowledged. Amy Kurtz writes with honesty and great compassion, helping readers feel less alone in their experience. Her words offer understanding, reassurance, and a sense of being met—like a trusted presence walking alongside you."

—TARA BRACH, AUTHOR OF *RADICAL ACCEPTANCE* AND *TRUSTING THE GOLD*

"For so many, the fear of relapse can be a significant hurdle on the road to recovery. *But You* Look *Fine*, by Amy Kurtz, tackles this issue head-on, offering evidence-based strategies to manage anxiety and build resilience. I highly recommend this book to anyone affected by illness—patients and healthcare professionals alike."

—LINDSAY TULCHIN, PHD

BUT YOU *LOOK* FINE

Also by AMY KURTZ

Kicking Sick: Your Go-To Guide for Thriving with Chronic Health Conditions

BUT YOU *LOOK* FINE

TRAPPED IN THE HELL BETWEEN SICK AND WELL AND HOW TO BREAK FREE

AMY KURTZ

FOREWORD BY LEO GALLAND, MD

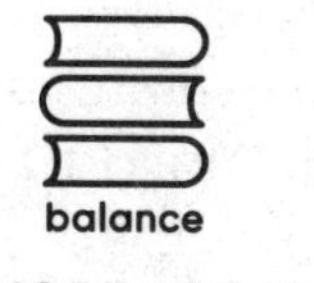

balance

NEW YORK BOSTON

The tools and information presented herein are not intended to replace the services of trained health professionals or be a substitute for medical advice. You are advised to consult with your health care professional with regard to matters relating to your health, and in particular regarding matters that may require diagnosis or medical attention.

Details relating to the author's life are reflected faithfully to the best of their ability, while recognizing that others who were present might recall things differently. Names and identifying details have been changed to protect the privacy and safety of others, including clients who shared their stories for this book.

Balance
Hachette Book Group
1290 Avenue of the Americas
New York, NY 10104
GCP-Balance.com
@GCPBalance

First Edition: June 2026

Balance is an imprint of Grand Central Publishing. The Balance name and logo are registered trademarks of Hachette Book Group, Inc.

The publisher is not responsible for websites (or their content) that are not owned by the publisher.

The Hachette Speakers Bureau provides a wide range of authors for speaking events. To find out more, go to hachettespeakersbureau.com or email HachetteSpeakers@hbgusa.com.

Balance books may be purchased in bulk for business, educational, or promotional use. For information, please contact your local bookseller or the Hachette Book Group Special Markets Department at special.markets@hbgusa.com.

Library of Congress Cataloging-in-Publication Data has been applied for.

ISBNs: 9781538775301 (Hardcover); 9781538775325 (ebook)

Printed in Canada

MRQ-T

10 9 8 7 6 5 4 3 2 1

To any patient who has felt
that they didn't have a voice,
this book is for you.

CONTENTS

Foreword by Leo Galland, MD xiii
Author's Note xvii
What's Wrong *with You?* xix

PART ONE: WHAT IS MEDICAL TRAUMA BRAIN?

1 The Shadowlands 1
2 Bumping Up Against Trauma 15
3 The Wild Ride of Fear Looping and the Three *E*s 31
4 All the Effing *F*s 49
5 The Wild, Wild Western Medical System 65
6 From the Passenger's Seat to the Driver's Seat 83

PART TWO: TOOLS FOR HEALING

7 Riding the Wave 101
8 Creating Space for Healing 119
9 No More Masks 147
10 Huddle Up! Becoming Your Own Health Coach . . . 167
11 Retrain Your Brain (-Body) 201
12 Safe Space 225

Conclusion 239
Acknowledgments 243
Notes 245
Index 259
About the Author 269

FOREWORD

Chronic illness has become part of the fabric of life in this country, impacting people of all ages and families of all types. Its growth has been driven by many factors: environmental, nutritional, infectious, and social. These external influences drive internal disharmony, disrupting the body's immune system, hormones, and neurotransmitters, and disrupting the microbiome, the trillions of microbes that naturally inhabit our bodies. For most people with chronic illness, there's not one cause or one solution, a fact that challenges the fundamental paradigm of modern Western medicine, which is that people get sick because they contract a disease.

I've specialized in treating patients with complex, chronic illness for the past forty-five years. "Complex" means that there's more than one problem; there are what scientists call "co-morbidities," different medical conditions co-existing in the same person, sometimes closely related to one another and sometimes not so clearly related. As the epidemic of complex, chronic illness has exploded over the past several decades, the number of co-morbid conditions has expanded and the people suffering from its reach have become younger and younger. When I started my medical career, chronic disease was understood as a geriatric problem, readily seen in the frailty of old age. As the epidemic has spread to younger people, there's been a dramatic increase of invisible illness, which is hard to measure and not obvious to an observer, even one with medical training.

Illness can change us and, when severe or chronic, can change our concept of who we are. We become *patients*, a term derived from the Latin verb *patior*, which means "to suffer." The suffering of illness extends beyond the physical symptoms. Perhaps the worst part is fear, not only fear of sickness, but fear of loss: the loss of identity, independence, valued relationships, and hopes for the future. Despite the substantial technological advances that have improved medical treatment over the past forty-five years, there has been no improvement in the ability of the health care system to alleviate this fear of loss. People who are sick have to navigate by themselves. Living with a chronic illness that others don't see can dramatically increase your suffering. When your illness is invisible to others, you are at risk of losing the support of family and friends that is so important to each of us in overcoming adversity. People with invisible illness often find that health professionals don't take them seriously. You may begin to doubt your own experience or get drawn into a vortex of hypervigilance, afraid that the wrong step will either make you sicker or expose you to the critical judgment of others. Tension between self-doubt and hypervigilance further amplifies the suffering, but denial and distraction are rarely helpful because illness can act like a screaming child that demands attention and forces you, over and over again, to confront the effects it has on your life.

I have worked with thousands of patients trapped in this way by invisible illness. They are looking for answers: What is wrong with me and what can be done to treat it? The answers to those questions are important, and my job, as a medical professional, is to help deliver them. Beyond that, what every patient needs is *agency*: knowledge of the steps you yourself can take to control illness, improve health, and overcome your suffering. Our medical system does nothing to enhance agency. In fact, it is structured to undermine it, especially for people with invisible illness. I have learned that supporting the agency of my patients is as important for their recovery as diagnosis and treatment.

Amy Kurtz has lived with a multifaceted, chronic, and invisible disease for most of her life and has spent years counseling other people with similar afflictions. In *But You* Look *Fine*, she dives deep into her experience as a patient and a helper to shed light on this essential and neglected aspect of healing. She shares her own story, the stories of friends and clients, and the wisdom she has received from some of the world's leading experts in overcoming emotional trauma. The vision and the synthesis are uniquely her own, as she guides her readers to an understanding of a condition she calls Medical Trauma Brain (MTB). Her point: that being chronically sick can create as much damage as physical trauma and can leave you with a post-traumatic stress disorder, even if you are recovering medically.

Amy's work is designed to help you understand the impact of illness on your emotions, your thoughts, and your relationships with the people who are important in your life. Her goal is to empower you to grow into agency through understanding the steps you need to take to gain control of your emotions, thoughts, and interactions with others, including health professionals, and to overcome self-destructive patterns of behavior. Because she has experienced firsthand the role of diet and environment in creating her own illness, she offers a practical approach to understand how you can gain agency by controlling the food you eat and the air you breathe.

If you or a loved one suffer from an invisible chronic illness, *But You* Look *Fine* is essential reading. Through its pages, Amy Kurtz presents a structured program that will immeasurably enhance your journey toward healing.

—Leo Galland, MD

AUTHOR'S NOTE

I'm so glad you're here. I promise to do my very best to help you navigate this world of confusion, isolation, anxiety, loneliness, and so many other feels that you're currently experiencing—this limbo between sick and well that I call *Medical Trauma Brain* (MTB).

I struggled for over a decade with a serious illness, which launched me into becoming a patient advocate and health coach. I worked with a very prominent physician and developed a health coaching program adjacent to his medical practice. Over time, I started hearing something over and over again from the patients and my private clients that I had never heard anywhere. It had never been named, and there was no language for it. In my own recovery, I didn't know what was happening inside myself either.

MTB is real. I know it, and I know you do, too. That's because we're living it. But because so few people know about MTB or understand what it is, up to this point there's been no real discussion about it. There's been no acknowledgment and no path to healing—until now!

Where this understanding comes from is not because I'm a doctor. I'm not. But I have lived it, researched it, worked with doctors on it, and this book is going to show you how to get through it.

What I share in this book are some of the tools that I have personally found to be helpful in managing and healing, along with approaches that my clients have found useful. I'm not trying to imply that every tool or methodology I'll discuss is going to be right for you. The information in this book is meant to serve as inspiration, not a prescription. (If you're anything like me, you've already had way too many of those!)

When it comes down to it, we're each unique. It requires a combination of self-awareness and exploration to discover what truly works *for you*. And that's what this book is all about: empowering you to connect with yourself on a deep level so you can make the choices that are best for you.

This journey you're about to take won't always be easy, but I'll be right here with you the whole time. And I've done my best to ensure that as you read and as you start on the path to healing, you'll be feeling some good vibes, too. Things like love, validation, support, and hope.

You ready to start taming that MTB monster, look it square in the face, and get the heck out of this limbo and into the bright sunny place? Let's go. I've got you. Take my hand.

Love,

Amy

WHAT'S *WRONG* WITH YOU?

I was only halfway through my Lyme disease treatments, but based on how well I was already feeling, it was evident that I was in for a major life change. Having been through so many cycles of illness and intervention in my life, I could tell that this was different. The end, and real healing, were in sight. I was doing it! But for some reason I wasn't clicking my heels and returning home. Despite being "better" on paper and feeling better than I had felt in a long time, something inside me still felt off. Rather than feeling care-free, I was embroiled in bouts of anxiety, and at one point even had a panic attack. But why?

You see, for most of my life, I've been struggling with chronic illness, so I'm no stranger to this roller-coaster. While I've certainly felt better without being "well," something was different here. My physical woes began at age fourteen when I became virtually debilitated by a hideous bout of chronic, very-long-term back pain. From that point forward, I was on a quest to feel better, bouncing from this treatment to that, including round after round of anti-inflammatories, but nothing seemed to help. And somehow I pressed on. In the years that followed, I did the best I could with what I had. I thought, *This is my new normal.* Then at twenty-five, during a trip abroad, I had a serious (and I mean serious) health crisis. There I was in the hospital, once-vibrant me now suddenly exhausted and languishing, a shell of my former high-energy, life-loving self. The situation felt chaotic and frightening, and once again the cause was a mystery.

My entire life came to a grinding halt with my health and healing becoming my entire focus because the situation demanded it be. Yet as long and hard as the struggle was, I kept seeing it as "only a pause." *The rug is just ripped out from under me, for now,* I thought. I was convinced that at some point my docs and I would find the key to unlock what was going on with me, and I'd bounce back and rejoin my life as an actress already in progress. In that time I did what pretty much everyone with a chronic illness does—I adapted, constantly adjusting what I viewed as normal, shifting my perceptions to somehow encompass the crazy intensity and roller-coaster of my experiences. It's like, we pivot, and pivot, and pivot again.

Over time I did start to feel better—enough so that I was able to write my first book, *Kicking Sick*. It was my love letter from my heart to people struggling with chronic disease and a guidebook for how to thrive through something that could otherwise be sidelining and totally life-defining.

But the truth was that I still wasn't healthy. I was just health*ier*, or so I thought. After my book came out, I started to feel really unwell again, and then I began to plummet, feeling even sicker than before. I started to question my diagnosis. So I took a deep breath and I packed up my hopes and my dreams for great health and lugged them along to my thirty-sixth doctor (you read that right). Finally, through a series of many, many tests, at long last I got the correct diagnosis of late-stage neurological Lyme disease. When the doctor told me, I knew with every fiber of my being it was true. From that moment on, I jumped in, cannonballing straight into a whole new pool of treatments and lifestyle changes—and I got better! Like, for real. Better than maybe I'd ever felt before in my entire life! *Good,* I thought. *Now I can un-pause and get back to my life!*

And then the pandemic hit with all its crazy-making what-the-fuckness. I started to feel more anxious and high strung, worrying about every little thing. But that made sense. After all, everyone was stressed out, right? I mean, a global pandemic will do that to you.

As the lockdowns continued, at one point our apartment building experienced a leak. The management company in their wise wisdom decided that the best way to address it was to open up a wall in our unit so that it could dry out from the inside. But when they broke through the wall, what was revealed was horror-movie terrifying—a massive colony of black mold had been living all *People Under the Stairs*—like behind our wall. The fact that the black mold had been there lurking, unseen, was bad and creepy enough, but the drywall had provided some degree of protection. Opening the wall unleashed the full fury, and my husband, Danny, and I experienced a massive toxic mold exposure.

Literally overnight I exploded with symptoms. I broke out so badly that my body lit up like the night sky in New Mexico, with constellations of hives covering my skin. I developed a steady wheeze and became allergic to anything with a scent or with any kind of chemicals in it. If I got near anything moldy, I'd explode in fits of uncontrollable coughing. Suddenly it felt like anything in the environment had the potential to set me off.

When I got checked out, the doctor said that the levels of mold on my test results were the highest he'd seen during his forty-year career. *Thanks, Doc! I love a gold star but not that kind.* He added environmental sensitivities and mast cell activation syndrome to my list of diagnoses(eseses). At that point, I was like, *Seriously, God, or whoever's out there, we're in the middle of a pandemic and now I'm allergic to my house? That's a low blow.*

Finally, Danny and I were able to exit Moldsville and move into a new apartment. In the process, though, I had to get rid of loads of my stuff because I'd become allergic to it: stuffed animals that had comforted me in childhood, a hat that had belonged to a beloved friend and former client who had since passed, all of my books, and essentially everything porous in my home. Relatively speaking, the clothes were no big deal, and I was fortunate enough to have the option of replacing them. And they didn't have any real sentimental value. But my baby book? That was cruel. I just couldn't bring myself to get rid of it. As I write this, it's sitting sealed up in a storage locker.

Fortunately, our new locale and detoxing helped me to feel better and symptoms began to dissipate. Like I mentioned earlier, at this point I was also halfway through my Lyme treatments, which were a massive game changer. My doctor had told me I would feel like I had a new body, and I sure did. I was back on track and feeling better than I ever had in my adult life. At least physically. But mentally and emotionally? Not so much.

I didn't understand what was going on. My body was so much better, so why wasn't I celebrating? Why was I still so *tense* all the time? Why did I feel this overwhelming sense of fear and dread?

It wasn't until my husband took me on the worst date ever that it hit me like a ton of bricks. Danny casually said, "Hey, I wanna say something to you that might be, well, a little provocative."

"Oh?" My eyebrows launched into my hairline. "Okay," I said, trying to sound calm. I quickly diverted my attention to my salmon, which I pretended to suddenly find extremely interesting.

One of the things I love most about Danny is that he always tells it to me like it is. At that moment, though, it felt like one of my least favorite qualities.

No, I told myself, sighing internally. *You can handle it.*

I looked back to Danny. "What is it?" I asked.

"Well, I always knew there'd be another phase for you with this. With your illness. It's like, I've been prepared for the other shoe to drop."

I looked at him blankly. He'd been thinking this *all along*?

"Other shoe?" I asked.

"Yeah," he said. "You have been through so much. I mean, you've been sick for over two decades. I always expected that there would be a part two. What you've experienced has been incredibly traumatic, you know?"

Boy, did I.

He went on. "But I think that now that you're feeling better physically, you'll be able to work on that other piece."

Other piece? It took a moment for what Danny was saying to sink in. That long-term illness hadn't just affected me physically, but also mentally.

That other shoe he'd mentioned? Well, it had just dropped. And it wasn't some cute little Louboutin, it was a big old camouflage Croc. CLUNK! Right there in the middle of the table.

I sat there stunned. The whole time I'd been sick I thought I'd been caring for myself, not just physically but holistically. There was a whole regimen of self-care I'd undertaken. I meditated, did yoga, ate healthy . . . basically all the things. I'd even written about it in my book. And hello, *ten years* of talk therapy! I thought I'd been working all of the angles together.

In the days and weeks that followed, as I continued to reflect on what Danny had said, the picture became clearer. After I'd started the Lyme treatments and was experiencing real relief, suddenly I had all this room on my mental plate. After all, I no longer had to spend most of my energy and attention trying to navigate life as a sick person. My routines didn't have to be quite so strict or regimented anymore. So why couldn't I calm the fuck down? Why was I still so high strung? I had become like the sick police, constantly monitoring for the slightest sign that my symptoms were returning. I'd see a red dot on my skin and hit the panic button. *I knew it. It's a hive! The treatment stopped working and I'm going to be allergic to everything again and we're going to have to throw everything out and find a new place and I'll be coughing and wheezing all the time, walking around with the Big Dipper right across my face! [pause] Oh, it's just a pen mark.*

Every little thing that could possibly signal that I was getting sick or that I may in some way be unsafe again, would send me to eleven. I even became convinced that the symptoms I'd experienced right after my return from my trip to Israel when I was twenty-five would resurface. The slightest twinge in my back would have me bracing for a flood of pain. I was like this overeager, overprotective, hypersensitive superhero showing up on the scene with her cape on backwards and crazy hair, glasses half off her face. I was Super Freak!

Danny was right—I wasn't the same as I'd been before. Something had changed within me and not in the good "Defying Gravity"–way. And it was something that would require work to repair. I realized then that in some ways, my healing journey was only just beginning.

I started doing research, poking around to see if I could find anything that named what I was experiencing. The anxiety, hypervigilance, overreacting, and generally acting like an overbearing control freak about anything that might remotely affect my health.

It was like my mental and emotional wiring had been, well, rewired. But I wasn't really finding anything that described these feelings. I mean, more than a decade of therapy and no one ever said anything about an anxiety problem.

I went back and spoke to some of my physicians, asking if this was a thing. "Oh, yeah," some of them said, "I've seen that." But no one had a name for this phantom illness, and no one had a solution. I'd been to *thirty-six* doctors and not one had ever told me I'd need to deal with the mental and emotional effects of my physical illness. That being sick in my body had made me sick in my head. Instead, I had to put it together for myself. The fact that all of the physical challenges I'd experienced, all of the lab tests and not knowing, the ups and downs, not to mention the terrible experiences with doctors and medical staff—all of it had been *traumatic.* That's the word Danny had used. This dude with no medical training who was simply a bystander on the front lines of my chronic illness had nailed it.

That's when it hit me like a Croc to the face: *Holy shit, I have Medical Trauma Brain!*

This was followed closely by a second thought: *Wait, what the fuck is Medical Trauma Brain?*

As the days went on and I contemplated my new self-diagnosis of a condition whose name I made up, I became more and more convinced of something: That if I had Medical Trauma Brain (MTB), I sure as heck wasn't the only one.

MEDICAL TRAUMA BRAIN

With this new idea in mind, I turned back to my research, talked to my doctor, and recounted countless conversations with friends, clients, and fellow veterans of chronic illness for the last five years. The patterns became clear.

I asked my Lyme doctor, if in his decades of practice, he'd seen anything like what I was experiencing. He confirmed that, while not known by any particular name, what I described was something he, too, had witnessed. As he characterized it, it's that patient who, even though their symptoms improve or even go away entirely, still isn't okay. For some reason, they're not acting like they're better. And as I realized firsthand, the reason was that we *aren't* all better. We still have another kind of healing left to do.

That's when I realized that "better" isn't even a destination, it's relative. That "sick" and "well" aren't a dichotomy. Society, though, has other ideas. We walk around with this idea that you're one or the other, leaving no space in between. But the fact is that it's a spectrum. And that vast gap in between sick and well? Well, that can feel like hell. It's the illness after the illness.

And that hell is a place most of us with a chronic or invisible illness, who have spent chunks of our lives dedicated to "healing," find ourselves in. It's just that no one is talking about it. Sure, there are rumblings among doctors and researchers and mental health practitioners here and there, but there's no real, visible understanding and awareness among patients that this phenomenon—Medical Trauma Brain—exists and how many of us it affects.

Well, you, guess what? It's other-shoe time for you, too. If you're reading this and any of it sounds familiar—the anxiety, the obsessive hypervigilance, the fear like a tidal wave that the worst is coming back, and the general all-around crazy—there's a good chance that you (or perhaps someone you love) also have Medical Trauma Brain. And I'm planting a flag in this godforsaken land so that all of the nearly 194 million Americans (that's more than 76 percent of adults!) struggling with chronic illness can escape the confusion, ignorance, and gaslighting and find true, deep healing.

And these numbers barely scratch the surface of the billions around the world who are dancing with the demon of prolonged, unpredictable illness.

Medical Trauma Brain, or MTB as I'll often refer to it, is a phenomenon that somehow has gone unrecognized in our modern health system, but it's a significant and very real phenomenon, and what I believe is the missing piece in our true healing journey. Just like other forms of lingering traumatic stress, it's an invisible wound and it needs healing. But I have some good news. While getting there isn't easy, *healing is possible*. And I am going to show you how. I've done the digging, read the research, been the guinea pig, and I've interviewed some of the top experts in trauma to understand what MTB is and how to move through it. The result is this book you're holding right now in your hands.

In part one, we're going to answer the first big question you probably have when you find yourself in the hell between sick and well: *What happened to me?* We're going to unpack exactly what this hellacious hell is all about—what it feels like and how you got here. First, we'll visit a place I call The Shadowlands to get a better picture of what Medical Trauma Brain is, in part by seeing the stories of others who are struggling just like you (and me).

Then we'll unpack the mechanisms of MTB—what trauma is, how and why certain experiences become traumatic while others don't, what makes the trauma we've experienced so unique, and how a medical system that's supposed to help us (and often does) can also hurt us. By the time you're done with part one, you'll have a full handle on how Medical Trauma Brain affects what's happening inside you, along with a heavy dose of validation. Because you're not imagining it, my friend. Something truly is wrong inside you, but we can make it right again. That that's what part two is all about!

In the second half of this book, we're going to focus on healing. I'm going to share all of the tools I've learned to help manage and process my MTB. We'll start off by creating a kind of emergency response kit: a set of tools you can use to dial down the intense stress or anxiety so you can manage those spikes and function from a more stable space. Then we'll dive into the longer-term work, starting with ways to deal with dysregulation and rewire your nervous system so you're not so prone to those big swings and you can start to feel more grounded within yourself. From there, I'll take you on a journey into self-health coaching, where we'll look at the massive number of things you can do *all on your own* to improve the quality of your health and your life and move past MTB.

But while the decisions you make for yourself form the core of your health, for some things we need help, so from there we'll turn to the professionals and the modalities that can be particularly useful for addressing the unique brand of trauma you're dealing with. After that, we'll explore the identity crisis many find themselves in, the one that comes from becoming a professional patient and missing out on huge pieces of your life. We're going to explore some new ways to engage with life so you're no longer staring after that cruise ship from the dock. Instead, you'll be building *your own boat* and sailing!

In this book I have done my level best to provide you with every bit of information, guidance, and support I can to help you get out of this hell and experience true wellness and true healing. And not just that, but to experience something even deeper and more meaningful: a sense of safety inside yourself.

As you travel this path, rest assured that I'm going to be with you every step of the way, and we're going to do this thing together. I've got you.

All aboard the healing train! First stop: The Shadowlands.

PART ONE

WHAT IS MEDICAL TRAUMA BRAIN?

ONE

THE SHADOWLANDS

There I was, me, myself, and my Medical Trauma Brain. I thought I was on the road to recovery. And I was, physically. But mentally and emotionally I was barely hanging on. In a strange way I'd kind of normalized what I was experiencing—all the anxiety and fear. I mean, doesn't *everyone* freak out at the sound of a power saw and immediately email the building owner, super, and manager and request full details on the construction, immediately convinced that any work could release more toxic mold and cause a complete reappearance of all the symptoms they've just spent all this time and energy (and money) finally getting under control? To be fair to myself, and to those of you who've experienced this kind of thing, chemical sensitivity is real.

Yet the thing is, that anxiety (and okay, abject terror) isn't just me being irrational or worked up. It's simply par for the course when you're living with MTB, or as I like to describe it, living in a place called The Shadowlands.

Imagine you're having dinner with friends. Everyone's chatting and laughing, catching up on the news and the gossip. And while you're sitting right there with them, smiling and chuckling along, in your mind you're a world away. It's like your body is out for tapas, but your brain is in purgatory, trapped in a giant, gusting sandstorm where there is no one else in sight and no way out.

That's The Shadowlands. It's like everyone around you is in the regular world, but you're living in the Upside Down on *Stranger Things*. You're in this place that looks familiar, only it's all dark and gray and there's this creepy ashy confetti blowing around. But, NBD, right? Because it's become your new normal, so you don't even realize the disconnect. Still, the signs are all around, like that vague sense of loneliness or isolation you sometimes feel even in a room full of people. Or the flood of worry that envelops you when that smallest thing happens that you fear could trigger your illness.

Over and over again, you buckle down and brace for impact even though it may never come. But the most fucked up thing is that it might, because it has before. And that's why we're in this place. The most stressful type of stress is when something is unpredictable. It's aptly named chronic unpredictable stress. The worst might happen, or it might not. There's no telling! As a result, you're completely off-kilter.

After Danny gave me the gentle tough love and I finally put together the puzzle pieces, my entire perspective shifted. I realized that the amount of stress and worry I was carrying every day was extreme, yet I'd been coping with tough stuff for so long that my baseline was totally off. If you're anything like me, what happens is that the conditions we learn to tolerate as normal are what others might characterize as extreme. Things like spending a part-time job's worth of hours juggling medical appointments, wrestling with insurance companies, trying to get a copy of your damn test results already, finding ways to tolerate dehumanizing and disparaging treatment by doctors and other medical staff, or daily sessions sitting on the bathroom floor with your head propped against the side of the toilet because your new meds cause Tilt-a-Whirl–level nausea.

I'd been living in survival mode for so long that it had become my home. But when I panned back, I realized that my house was on fire. Ironically, I finally felt good enough in some ways to realize how bad I felt in others.

First, I'd spent decades navigating the labyrinth of pain and illness (along with a medical system where doctors frequently dismiss patients, but we'll get to that later). Then, there was the pandemic, and we all remember what that was like. On top of that, the mold exposure. When it comes to your experiences, I bet you have your own Jenga tower of doom. Maybe on top of chronic illness (along with a drastically diminished bank account thanks to all the bucks you spent to simply get well), your stress has been compounded by other life issues, like the loss of a job, challenges with your kids, and so on. The options are endless. The point is that when you're living in The Shadowlands, you're ill-equipped to deal with these issues, but life just keeps a'stackin'. Eventually, that tower can start to get reeeeal wobbly, and may even crash.

Yet here's one of the things that's so tough about all of that. As someone coping with a chronic illness and all that it brings with it, you've probably gotten really good at dealing with challenges. When stuff goes south, you pull up your britches, take a deep breath, and do what needs to be done. You get the next round of tests. Commit to the extreme juice diet. Or take the medication with the terrible side effects. That's how you've made it this far: intense hypervigilance and being regimented to get better as soon as possible. You've learned how to normalize some crazy stuff to keep it together and do what needs doing, all in the hopes that at some point, you'll pop out on the other side of the long, dark tunnel.

In fact, you can get so clutch at coping that at times, it can come as a surprise just how okay you're *not* doing.

In The Shadowlands your ability to manage is maxxed out like a college credit card, but you don't necessarily realize it until your purchases start getting declined. It's when something happens and you try to shift into management mode, but you find that suddenly you just don't have that gear. It's simply not in you to manage One. More. Thing. It's like what happened to me a while back when I got a call from my compounding pharmacy.

SPIRALING

Every month for the last ten years, the very same angel at my compounding pharmacy had been mixing up her special recipe for my thyroid medicine. I started on a compounded medication because the regular drugs my old endocrinologist gave me for my hypothyroidism were just too much and I ended up with thyroid toxicosis, which is exactly as fun as it sounds. Picture your heart pounding so hard and fast you're afraid your chest is going to burst open like a crew member from the *Nostromo* in *Alien*. I was gasping for air, feeling like I couldn't take a breath, sweating like crazy. Needless to say I changed endocrinologists, then after the acute portion of this particular picnic was over, spent the next year slowly weaning my way down on dosage as my body detoxed.

If you have thyroid issues, you know what an enormous deal they are. Your endocrine system affects essentially everything else in your body, so when your thyroid is off, it can have a global impact on your health. The point is, having the right kind and dosage of medication is extremely important.

A little while back, out of the blue, I got a call from the manager at my pharmacy. "Hi there, Amy. It's Joe Schmo. Yeah, hey, I just wanted to let you know that your pharmacist won't be doing compounding anymore, effective, like, *now*, so you'll have to find a new pharmacy right away. And, we don't have any more of your medicine so we can't mix you an interim dose. Okay? Good luck!"

I sputtered. I think my mouth was literally hanging open. In total shock and panic, before he could hang up, I blurted out, "I need to talk to Sally!" the pharmacist in question.

"Oh, yeah, well, you can't," Joe said. "She doesn't want to talk to *you*."

What? Doesn't want to talk to me? That made no sense at all. I'd always had a great relationship with Sally. Hadn't I? It was confusion on top of the mayhem that was going off in my mind. *What's going on with Sally? Why is she leaving? How can Joe be such an ass?* And most important, *How the hell am I going to get my meds?!* It was a full-scale freakout. Inside I'd rocketed straight into survival mode, and all of the shmo shit, the condescension, and the chaos got shelved for later.

It wasn't until a week later—after I'd secured a new pharmacy and after Sally, herself, had called to apologize for Joe's schmo-ery, tell me the full story of their professional breakup, and help me get squared away—that I began to process what had happened. How when Joe called, I'd felt betrayed, belittled, abandoned, invalidated. The list goes on. But when I started to process all of this, I realized something else. Processing feelings post-stress is kind of a new thing for me. Most of the time I'd struggled with illness, I'd just push those feelings down and move on to the next thing. And that's a common pattern with chronic illness.

Raise your hand and gimme an amen if this has ever happened to you. You have an emergency—a flare up, a scary test result, an insane side effect from a new medication—and your emotions spike. Only you don't have time for those because you've got to take care of business and get your health in order. So, you put them on a shelf and focus on figuring out next steps.

If you're lucky, the issue is resolved, or you somehow make your way through it. But then . . . nothing. Often there's no processing of that insane survival stress you experienced because we're in a system that doesn't recognize that sick people have *feelings* about what happens to us. Plus, we live in a culture that prizes the ability to soldier on through tough times over emotional caretaking and a well-regulated nervous system. Since no one talks about these things—about processing traumatic events—we move on. And then it happens again. And again. Fast-forward into the future and hello, Medical Trauma Brain! And hello, Shadowlands.

POSTCARDS FROM THE SHADOWLANDS

Sadly, I have a lot of company in The Shadowlands. A few weeks ago, I was doing a podcast interview for a show on Lyme disease, and as part of my preparation I listened to some past episodes. Guest after guest, along with the hosts, described the various mental and emotional challenges they were experiencing, and it was obvious to me that they were reporting live from the heart of The Shadowlands. They all talked about their fear of the disease coming back, the inability to "move on," and so on. Yet there was no name for what they were experiencing and no definition. It was all vague, but because of my revelation I could see it all so clearly.

As I started thinking about this book and set out to prove my theory about MTB right, I approached some people I know who've dealt with chronic medical conditions and asked them to share some of their experiences. One—we'll call her Maggie—suffered with debilitating migraines for most of her life. Then, a few years ago, she started getting them nearly every day, *for over three years*!

"At first everyone was caring and sympathetic," Maggie told me, "but eventually it became so repetitive that people just kind of walked around me as I was lying there on the couch with a cold compress on my head and tears rolling down my cheeks. I felt like a piece of furniture. Even when I told doctors about the frequency and severity of my headaches, they barely responded. It was like they didn't believe me."

Then she spent a year working with a doctor who failed to help her at all. "I had three-hundred-thirteen migraines I didn't need to have because of her!" Maggie said. Finally, fortunately, like me she found a doctor who could help and she's doing much better now. But looking back on that time when her migraines were so persistent is painful for her.

Then Maggie said something to me that flat-out floored me. "When I fully grasped what you were saying—that the residual trauma caused by the chronic illness was just as real as the illness itself—a lightbulb went off for me. I realized that at this point, I've been suffering more from the trauma than the migraines. But more importantly, for the first time in years, I realized I no longer have chronic migraines!" As she explained, even when she was feeling fine, she'd always assumed that the next migraine was just around the corner, and that anything could trigger it. She'd been so fixated on this idea that she failed to realize how rare it had become for her to actually have a headache. This is how The Shadowlands obscures our thinking. Maggie was more focused on her fear and anxiety than actual symptoms.

Another woman, whom I'll call Lori, shared that after decades trying to get her Lyme under control, she started to notice other issues. Once she started feeling better physically, she felt a kind of depression set in. It was like the world expected her to just get on with her life, but she needed time to recover mentally—to recalibrate—but culturally we don't do that. We don't have that concept. "It started to sink in that I've spent most of my adult life being a patient, and now I have a new kind of stress. I have to play catch-up with all of the other people my age who got to start a career in their early twenties instead of being in the hospital. I'm so grateful that I'm feeling better now, but it's like I have to use all of my energy trying to figure out the rest of my life because I'm starting from behind."

Lori also echoed Maggie's sentiment that a lot of people just don't know what to do with someone who is or has been so sick. They don't have a context for it or don't have the emotional capacity to be compassionate or to connect with you. And so your social circle can shrink, along with your romantic life. Even family can pull back. When you're finally able to get back out there and start trying to build new relationships, it's scary. Should you share what you've been through? Will that scare people off? Gang, I hear you—I've been there, too.

For Lori's part, she moved to a new city to try a start fresh. She told me about a dinner she went to with some new acquaintances. When the waiter put a glass of wine down in front of her, the other women at the table didn't realize what a momentous occasion it was for Lori. Due to her health struggles, she hadn't had a drop of alcohol in seven years. She decided to share but didn't get the reaction she was hoping for. Instead of something that looked like understanding or compassion, the girls erupted into *Whoop-whoops* and high fives. "Party!" they shouted. Instead of seen, Lori felt even more isolated. It reinforced the "I'm not like other people" meme that had been playing in her mind.

But here's the thing. Just like Maggie, Lori didn't totally really realize she was experiencing all of this until we spoke about it. Of course she had some awareness, but my description of MTB got her to step back and really think about what she was experiencing.

I just want to zoom back in here on that idea of bracing for impact. See how Maggie experiences all that stress just from anticipating that a migraine *might* set in? For me, it's the first indication of what could be a Lyme flare. For someone with rheumatoid arthritis, it could be a twinge of joint pain that sets the stress machine in motion.

I'm going to hit a pause button here and address you directly, Dear Reader. Let's make room for some of the feels you might be feeling right about now. Perhaps you're realizing some things for the first time, too. Maybe you're not even totally aware of it, but your body could be telling you. Take a few moments and just check in. Take a deep breath and notice how you're feeling. What's going on in your mind? What are you feeling in your body? In your heart? Maybe get up and do a little stretch or take a sip of water. Pull out your journal or phone a friend if you need to. Take your time. I'll be here.

I just want to encourage you to be gentle with yourself and to check in periodically to notice how you're feeling. Because this stuff we're talking about? It's big.

Suffice it to say, MTB is real and so are the ways it impacts us. So, let's take a closer look at what it is and why it develops.

THE ROOTS OF MTB

From chronic illness to acute injuries, medical issues are stressful. That stress, whether immediate, intense, and short-lived or more variable and prolonged, can be traumatic. That's because serious medical issues put us into survival mode—that place where we believe that we're fighting for our life and may actually be—so we experience something trauma experts call *survival stress*.

We'll get into some of the physiological and psychological details of trauma in the next chapter, but for now, here's what you need to know: In some cases, we can and do process and release survival stress relatively quickly. Humans are actually amazingly resilient. But in many cases, we don't. Or we don't process and release all of it. When we've got unprocessed survival stress it doesn't just magically evaporate. Instead, it cozies up and makes a home deep down inside us, becoming *stored survival stress*, a.k.a. trauma. Add to that the ongoing deposits we're making to this unfortunate account as our survival stress continues, because that's life with ongoing illness. And yet again, as common as this is, it's almost never called out by medical providers, which is just another way the system fails people with chronic illness.

So why call it out as Medical Trauma Brain, specifically, and not just say "trauma"? Well, a few reasons. For starters, trauma is a really broad term, and these days it's used so easily as to be nearly meaningless in some cases. But more important, calling and framing out MTB as trauma related to experiences with chronic illness and the medical system helps us more easily identify that we have it. And when we know we have it, we can start to address it.

As I mentioned before, when I talked to everyone from doctors to folks with chronic illness, although everyone got the concept of MTB, it was essentially a news flash for all of them. Like, "Oh, yeah, now that you mention it . . ." Creating awareness around lasting medical trauma is essential because you can't heal what you don't know you have. On top of that, hopefully this whole discussion will bring more awareness to those in the medical system who are contributing to or even causing some of this trauma. (I'm lookin' at you, Joe.)

To help you get a better handle on Medical Trauma Brain and how and why it develops, I've isolated six phases of the chronic illness experience that can contribute to MTB. See if you recognize them. To be clear, not everyone who has these experiences develops MTB, but if you have MTB, then you'll probably recognize most or all of them.

One: WTF?

First, there's the sheer confusion of feeling sick and not knowing what's wrong. It's deeply ungrounding, to say the least. It's like your entire life axis shifts and your focus narrows and becomes centered around survival because *it has to.*

Two: The Diagnosis

Then comes the diagnosis, which can feel like a life sentence and lead to all sorts of painful questions. Or, the diagnosis might not be definitive. The doctor might only have a sense of what's indicated by your symptoms and test results rather than a clear picture. So, on one hand it can feel like you're locked in a prison by a diagnosis, or it can be more like you're floating in space, hoping to gain more clarity so you at least know for sure what it is you're dealing with.

Three: Identity Shift

In an act of self-preservation, you transition into becoming a "Sick Person." A portion of your life is taken over. For the longest time when I looked back on my life, it was like I was two people. First, I was a kid, and then I was a kid in pain. There's a before and an after, and in many ways it feels like the old you is gone forever, replaced by this new identity: Lyme patient, Crohn's patient, Lupus patient. It's how we see ourselves and how the medical system sees us: as a patient who needs fixing. It's often in this stage that you realize that you're in it for the long haul—that tending to your health is essentially your new part-time, or even full-time, job.

Four: Treatment Hell

Treatments often make us feel worse before we feel better, adding another layer of frustration. On top of that there's another emotion—something that's more profound. It's a form of grief.

What has your life come to? Another common part of Treatment Hell is the "Let's try *this*!" approach where doctors aren't sure what will help, so they run a million tests, then start you on a litany of meds hoping that one will be the magic pill. When you have an invisible or ongoing illness that doesn't have a clear solution, sometimes the very person who's supposed to be able to help you is struggling to do just that. This often results in you as the patient feeling like you can't let up—you have to have your own back and advocate for yourself to the point of exhaustion.

As each new treatment begins, you're twiddling your thumbs, waiting to see if it works. You may feel so bad and so panicked that you can end up in desperation mode where you're willing to try just about anything. "Wait, this stuff turns your skin purple and makes your mouth go numb? Okay, never mind, I'll do it!" And then if you do find something that works, you're apparently on it forever. Rarely is there talk of getting you off or trying to transition to non-pharmaceutical approaches.

Five: Isolation

All of this lands us in a place of isolation. No one else seems to understand the nature of the craziness we're going through. We feel misunderstood by people around us, neglected by loved ones and society, and are often expected to just deal with it. The even bigger problem is that the medical system itself compounds the issue by not acknowledging the damage that a chronic illness does to your identity and your psyche. Doctors tend to just put a label on a patient's physical symptoms. They diagnose and treat the illness but are often insensitive and ineffective at dealing with the effects of the illness. To be fair, they're generally not trained in this, but that's a serious problem in and of itself, as we'll discuss later.

Six: The Hamster Wheel

You find yourself on a hamster wheel of desperation, trying to find the right doctor, diagnosis, and treatment to feel better, not stopping no matter how fast you have to run. Eventually, it becomes more about the *fear* of being sick, and you feel like you're stuck on that wheel, afraid the whole awful cycle will start again. At some moments you can feel totally disoriented, like you don't even know where you are in your treatment journey. How long are you supposed to hang out in this space or chug around that damn wheel? And how are you ever supposed to get off it and move on when there's no help or guidance?

Again, just like Kübler-Ross's stages of grief or Maslow's hierarchy of needs, these experiences aren't necessarily sequential. You can bounce back and forth among them, and you can also experience multiple phases at the same time.

The point is, these phases of chronic illness contribute to Medical Trauma Brain and the feeling of being in The Shadowlands.

While MTB is a new thing by name, some researchers and clinicians have been poking at its edges for a while. In the next chapter, we'll look at some of the research on medical trauma and how it relates to MTB. We'll also take a deeper look at how survival stress turns into lasting trauma.

TWO

BUMPING UP AGAINST TRAUMA

Back at that fateful dinner, when Danny first used the T-word with me, it was hard to wrap my mind around it. Trauma? *Really?* But the more I reflected on it, and the more I read about it, the more I realized how right he was.

In the last chapter, we explored the concept of The Shadowlands, which is my name for the *experience* of Medical Trauma Brain. Now, we're going to start unpacking the *mechanisms* of MTB, including some of the general science around trauma and how it ties in with chronic illness.

First, let's hit rewind for a minute. Remember in the last chapter how we talked about that idea of putting our emotions and our mental reactions on a shelf? It's like your hands—and your brain—are totally full trying to deal with the issue. You're attempting to get an accurate diagnosis, you're trying out a whole plethora of medications hoping something does the trick, you're following up on that referral to (yet another) specialist.

In all of this, you could be encountering some pretty lousy behavior on the part of doctors, medical staff, and sometimes even well-meaning friends, family, or co-workers. But you don't have time for that now! And you don't have time to address your *feelings* about any of what's happening because you're too busy trying to not die or become permanently disabled. Or you're just trying to claw your way back from the depths.

You're having all these reactions, and you're experiencing all of this stress, but there's nowhere to really go with it. For people with chronic illness, that's just part of the deal. Something happens—a new symptom, another test, a new med—it sucks, and then you move on. There's no time or opportunity to effectively process your thoughts and emotions about your experiences, plus—if you're like I was—you may not even be aware that's a thing. That chronic illness and our life as a perpetual patient can be *seriously traumatic*. And over time, that trauma compounds.

I think of it like that episode of *Friends* where the gang discovers that compulsive perfectionist Monica has a secret storage closet. When they finally wrench it open, they discover that it's crammed-to-bursting with all her shit, just threatening to explode all over the place. That's what's going on in our mental closet when we have MTB, only we're often not aware of it. It's like, even *we* don't know we have that closet, but all along we've been stuffing our feelings, our fear, and our anxiety into it so we could focus on the priority, which is trying to get better. Or maybe we're aware of it, but we just don't have the time or energy to open that door and go all Marie Kondo on our emotional clutter.

As we'll explore later in the book, the problem isn't just lack of awareness, it's lack of language. We don't have the words or the reference points to describe what we're experiencing, so it goes unacknowledged and the feelings keep building up. All of this starts to take up more and more of our mental and emotional bandwidth and we have less available to deal with life—whether it's the big stuff like illness or even just the mundane stuff. When you're dramatically under-resourced, just discovering that the sink is clogged could set you into a full-blown collapse.

That's the sad irony. While we may, in fact, be getting better physically, our emotional and mental suffering may be intensifying because there is finally more space for it. And as we'll explore later, that mental pain can contribute to or create more physical issues. But at the time the stress is happening, we're not worried about that. In the moment we're focused on being a *good patient*, on being a *warrior*, and on beating this thing. We're focused on being *resilient*. But while resilience is powerful, it can have a downside.

THE RESILIENCE TRAP

Resilience is often presented like it's a psychological panacea. Meaning, as long as you're resilient, you can withstand essentially anything that happens and just bounce back. It's like you're an action hero casually putting on your sunglasses as you walk off, like, "Oh, did a huge building just explode right behind me? I didn't even notice because I'm so damn resilient."

Resilience is the hallmark of being a good patient, and that's largely because of how we view resilience culturally. The gold stars go to the patients who are tough. The fighters. The ones who put their heads down, don't complain, and get on with the work of healing.

Good patients don't have emotional breakdowns. We don't question our doctor when a course of treatment they're advising doesn't make sense to us. We don't even ask too many questions, period.

Broadly speaking, I think this is more common for women. We tend to grow up with this ideal of the "good girl" who doesn't upset people and doesn't cause too much of a fuss. When we get into the doctor's office, we translate good girl into good patient. The whole rigamarole of chronic illness can weigh on us even more because it's so *inconvenient*, and in our society being inconvenient or being "hysterical" are two of the worst sins a woman can commit.

True story: An acquaintance who's a doctor once advised me specifically not to "get too emotional" in the doctor's office because it could potentially distract the doctor from the important business of treating me. To be fair, this person was simply expressing an idea that's largely assumed to be true: that feelings are messy and inconvenient and have nothing to do with patient "care." That the best patients suck it up, put their heads down, and get on with it. They were actually trying to help me get an accurate diagnosis and were afraid my emotions might cloud the doctor's opinion.

And get this. In my first book, *Kicking Sick*, I even advised readers to do the same! I had a whole section about how to be a good patient, which included not getting overly emotional and other tips and tricks to ensure you're making the most of your doctor's precious time. Gang, this stuff goes *deep*. It's taken me a long time to unlearn the good patient schtick, and I'm still working on it (in chapter 6 we'll look at some healthier, yet still constructive, ways to relate to your doc).

Sadly, to some extent this person was right in what they said—the part where showing emotion could short-circuit the doctor's judgment. Often when I did allow myself to share my feelings during an appointment, inevitably the doctor's eyes would glaze over. I could almost see the thought bubble floating next to their head. *Oh, I see the problem—she's hysterical.* One doctor even went so far as to suggest that my myriad ongoing symptoms would be resolved by a prescription of Xanax (I wish I was joking).

Don't get me wrong, resilience is a remarkable and at times lifesaving tool, and it's one we want to possess. There are moments when you need to be able to take that deep breath and do the hard thing. To keep calm and carry on! But like all tools, it can cause harm if it's misused. And I would venture to say that a healthier definition of resilience would include the ability to process our emotions.

It's true that when we're dealing with a chronic illness we don't want to collapse into a sobbing, snotty mess at every turn. Some part of us has to be able to keep moving forward. But when it's overused, resilience can become a way to bypass the truth of our situation, how much it sucks, and the toll it takes on us. When chronic resilience is what's demanded of us, or we impose that demand on ourselves, we pay a steep price. That price is MTB.

I know someone who fell and broke her jaw *and* she had heart surgery. She came home from the hospital with her jaw wired shut and instead of curling up on the couch and resting, *she made and hosted a Thanksgiving dinner*! I kid you not. She was acting like she was going for gold in the Good Patient Olympics, pushing through it all, almost pretending that her health issues just weren't happening. The reality is that bones don't just heal with the snap of a finger. After several weeks of toughing it out, she finally backed off, admitting that she was frightened and overwhelmed. She had to step away from the chronic resilience posture because her body just hurt too much. Now she accepts that when she hurts, she is actually really hurting, and that it's okay because that's part of the healing process.

I know that idea sounds kind of basic, but how often have you not listened to a call inside yourself to back off and be gentle? The reality is that we don't celebrate that behavior, and we need to start. Otherwise, we're constantly resisting our real feelings by saying "I can cope, I am fine!" And in this, we lose touch with our own voice and our own feelings. Acceptance enters the ring when we decide to step out of the Illness Olympics. In our culture we're taught to barrel through and not make anything more complicated or make anyone else feel bad. But what does that do to us and our recovery? First, we must stop prioritizing other people's reactions to our illness. Our reaction matters. We have to stop dismissing our own bodies and our own feelings. Typically, we accept what someone else tells us instead of being our own best advisor and caretaker, and we need to shift that.

Earlier in the book, I mentioned how people who are chronically ill assume the identity of "Sick Person," and this resilience thing is actually part of how we start to lose ourselves. We stop listening to the voice inside us that says things like, "That doesn't feel right," or "I think we need to take it easy today." Instead, we assume that some external authority—a doctor, a nurse, another person with the same illness, the health magazine we just read while we were getting our infusion—must know better than us so we should mute our own voice and do what they say.

The other side to this coin is that it's okay to not be okay. It's okay to be exhausted. Once we start to accept where we are and surrender to it, we'll gradually start to feel less threatened because we have mentally acknowledged that we need to give ourselves some space. It's okay to hurt and surrender to the fact that wounds take time to heal, as does the aftermath of being sick. In fact, the combination of dealing with chronic illness, along with doing our best to be a perfect patient, can create its own wound—the invisible wound of trauma.

WAKING UP TO TRAUMA

When we're sick, we press on through a massive amount of pain and suffering because we're focused on getting better and don't really have another choice. We simply don't have the bandwidth available to process our emotions around it. This plants the seeds for future trauma—seeds that often don't sprout and grow until we start to feel better.

Healing from something that's acutely painful, like fibromyalgia or scleroderma; dealing with an illness where the very "cure" requires great strength to endure, like chemotherapy for cancer or surgery for Crohn's disease or endometriosis; or confronting a mystery illness that evades diagnosis and defies attempts to treat it (hi, Lymies!)—all of these require a tremendous amount of energy as patients. And their ongoing nature means that for long periods of time, we are stuck in literal survival mode. If, on top of that, we get into a pattern of ignoring our feelings and suppressing our inner voice, we can compound the stress we're already experiencing from being sick.

If you're anything like me, while all of this is going on, you're just doing your damnedest to keep it together. When the waves—or the tsunami—hit, you're trying to hold on and not get sucked under. Then comes another wave, and another, so you grip harder and hang on and keep paddling, hoping that the shore will eventually materialize or the water will become shallow enough so at least you can stand. While you're fighting for your life, there's no time or space to process how you feel about all of it. So being both sick and *dealing* with that sickness—being resilient—can each be traumatic in their own ways.

I dealt with chronic illness for so long but lived in survival mode even longer. As a result, I lost my baseline, and when you've got no grounding, it's impossible to thrive. Plus, I lost something along the way. When my Lyme disease treatments started to work, it was like I came back to life, but it wasn't exactly *my* life. It was like at age twenty-five some part of me had gone to sleep, then when I woke up, I was thirty-nine. Fourteen years lost in the tidal wave of chronic illness. This is a personal tragedy so many of us with chronic illness share. Remember my friend Lori in chapter 1 talking about how she felt like she was so far behind her peers, just starting out on her career when everyone else had been at it for a decade or more?

Once we finally come up for air, once that shore is finally in sight, once our toes finally touch the sand, we may no longer be sick. Or our symptoms have at least diminished enough that we don't think we're in survival mode anymore. Part of our brain might be totally aware of that, and absolutely thrilled about it. The problem is, no one delivers that message to the rest of ourselves—to our bodies and those other parts of our brain where things got stuffed down. So deep inside, some part of us is still in survival mode. We're still fighting a perceived battle.

It's like that wild story about a Japanese soldier who'd fought in World War II and was discovered in the Philippines nearly three decades after the war. Only he wasn't sitting on the beaches drinking mai tais, he was still fighting. That's because *he didn't believe the war was over.* And here's the other dimension of that. The reason no one came and retrieved the soldier was that no one realized he was still there fighting! How's that for an apt metaphor? The battle with chronic illness is over (or at least greatly diminished), and we're starting to feel better, but we don't realize that some part of ourselves didn't get the memo *and is still fighting.* It's still anticipating, bracing, or reacting.

Long after we start to recover physically, we may suffer a psychic wound from having been sick for so long, and from everything we went through along the way. For me, even though I was "better," I couldn't get out of survival mode. I couldn't release my grip on resilience.

Why does a migraine sufferer still feel sick after the headaches have stopped? Why does a cancer patient still lose sleep for weeks after a scan even though they've gotten the "all clear"? That, my dear friends, is trauma. To be precise, it's Medical Trauma Brain.

To better understand how MTB came to be, let's put on our lab coats and have a little science lesson.

HOW SURVIVAL STRESS TURNS INTO TRAUMA

All of us experience trauma at some point in our lives, no matter what our circumstances. There's financial or food insecurity, loss, abuse, racism, and all the -isms and phobias. The list goes on. Those are just things we classically think of as traumatic, but the reality is that virtually anything can potentially cause trauma based on how we experience it. And we may also experience events that are completely harrowing but don't actually cause lasting trauma. Humans are complex, and each of us is so different that it's difficult to pinpoint exactly how certain circumstances or experiences will impact us.

The fact is that any time we experience survival stress—where we fear for our lives—there's the potential to experience trauma. And having a chronic illness and worrying that you'll actually die or get so sick that you'll never fully recover? That's about as survival-stressy as it gets. Only our good friend resilience tends to cloud this awareness. We're not sitting on the exam room table in a scratchy cotton gown with a paper blanket bunched up on our lap thinking, *Boy, I'm really experiencing some survival stress at this moment. I'm gonna need some support to process this shit out.*

No, we're thinking, *When's the doctor coming in? I've been waiting for forty minutes. Are my test results that bad? Is she thinking about how to break it to me? DEAR GOD, AM I DYING?!* Then we see the doorknob turn and we take a breath. *Okay, be cool. You can do this.* In other words, we put on our Good Patient mask by armoring up and engaging our resilience.

That's not a bad thing. I want to be super clear that I'm not judging that behavior. How could I judge it when that was me, always striving to be the best patient I could? Again, it's incredibly important to be able to handle some majorly tough stuff when you're dealing with a chronic illness. The point is, afterwards, you get off that table, put some real clothes on, and then step out the door and back into the rest of your life. You grab a coffee, phone a friend, finish your to-do list. Basically you're off to the races. Yet that survival stress you felt just an hour ago is still swirling and surging around inside you, even if you don't realize it. Then later, when something bumps up against it, you can get triggered. All the fear, anxiety, worry, or even anger flare up, but you're not sure why. Why does your reaction seem outsized to whatever just happened?

Have you ever had that experience where you bumped into something—maybe you hit your toe—and immediately you're hopping around yowling and holding your foot. Only three seconds later, you realize it didn't actually hurt, you're just reacting to the *memory* of pain from a time when you stubbed your toe and it was excruciating. Something inside you got all geared up because of an expectation your brain-body had. (Just a little note: I use "brain-body" here because while we often make a distinction between our brain and our body, they're interrelated in such complex ways—ways even our best and brightest scientists have yet to fully comprehend—that especially when it comes to our nervous system and trauma, it can be kinda' ridiculous to talk about them like they're totally separate entities.)

The point is, when you have MTB, which is all about the stress that lingers on inside us post-trauma, even when you feel or sense a ripple of something, it can feel like a tsunami. Suddenly, you're bracing for it. You get all amped up. Or for some it may be the opposite: you may go more into shut-down mode or numb out. These are both responses to when your nervous system is flooded with survival stress (Heads up: We'll discuss different types of reactions in more detail in chapter 4).

The total lack of predictability of a chronic illness, not knowing when the next wave is coming or even whether it will be a wave or a full-blown tsunami, is essentially the worst kind of stress there is because it's the hardest to process. That feeling of having no control or lacking any kind of certainty about your life, health, or what's coming next is horrible. Now imagine that experience extending over months, years, and even decades. *It's friggin' traumatic!* And when you start to feel better, that trauma doesn't just magically resolve itself (If only!).

That trauma can play out in a lot of ways. Those outsized reactions I described a moment ago can happen even when the event that triggers them seems to bear little resemblance to the original stressor. For instance, say one day you're getting on an elevator and as the doors close you start to have a panic attack. The sense of feeling closed in bumped into the extreme stress you felt while getting a CAT scan. Or maybe you're talking to your partner about what to do on date night. They're pushing hard for a movie even though you've already said you don't feel like it. Suddenly you're yelling at them. The feeling of not being listened to recalled your unexpressed anger at countless doctors who were dismissive toward you. You see how it works.

Yet here's the thing: *No one talks about this shit!* You know what would be amazing? If any one of those countless doctors you're seeing would stop and say, "Hey, you know, there's such a thing as 'survival stress' and at some point when you're ready and have the resources, you might want to get some help with that aspect of this experience." But they don't. Because they're likely not trauma informed, or they don't want to go there because it's too messy, and since they only have ten minutes to see you, there just isn't time. Instead, they'd rather we stay in Good Patient mode and *keep being resilient*, not recognizing that emotional processing is actually part of healthy resiliency.

In our culture it's a huge compliment to be called *resilient*, *tough*, or as I've been described over and over and over again, *tenacious*. But people never say stuff like, "She's a beast at processing difficult feelings!" or "Damn, that dude is emotionally agile." Ideally, we'd have some measure of both—the ability to meet the moment and the ability to go home afterwards and feel, name, and process all the difficult shit that we just went through. To me, that's how resilience should actually look. But as it is, we never get to that last part, so all that survival stress stays unresolved and trapped inside us, where it rewires our circuits.

In his book *The Trauma Spectrum*, Dr. Robert Scaer describes what happens this way: "In unresolved traumatic stress, procedural memory turns inward, responding to internal cues of a threat that no longer exists, evoking inappropriate somatic and autonomic experiences and responses that pertain to cues unwittingly emerging from past memory rather than from present external experiences." So, when we experience survival stress and we don't have a way to recognize and process it at the time, our procedural memories—a form of long-term memory that helps us learn how to do things automatically—can go haywire.

With MTB, we start to respond automatically to anything our brain-body decides could signal a threat, including normal, everyday things. Subtle signals set off massive alarms. For me, that could be the sound of hammering in my neighbor's apartment. My brain-body automatically decides that I might soon be exposed to a bunch of toxins, and the next thing I know, I'm in panic mode and doing damage control.

The etymological roots of the word "trauma" are in the ancient Greek, meaning "a wound, a hurt, a defeat." In *The Myth of Normal*, author and trauma expert Gabor Maté explains that trauma "is not what happens *to* you; it is what happens *inside* you as a result of what happens to you." He writes, "It is our woundedness, or how we cope with it, that dictates much of our behavior, shapes our social habits, and informs our ways of thinking about the world."

In other words, MTB is not about your illness, but what you experienced emotionally and mentally as a result. The more I started paying attention to this idea, the more places I saw it at work—in myself, in my clients, in my friends, pretty much everywhere. There is a common post-traumatic stress response that many of us have to ongoing illness, but it goes largely unnamed and undiscussed. But that changes now.

Hey, are you still with me? Or are you glazing over right about now? If so, give yourself a little pinch and stay with me! We're spending time on the science stuff because it'll be important for when we talk about how to begin to unwind all this trauma.

Also, not-so-fun fact: Going fuzzy or numbing out when we get into difficult details can be a trauma response. So, if you're feeling hazy, agitated, strung out—anything that signals you're off-kilter—take a breath. Maybe get yourself some water or even step outside and take a breath of fresh air. Or you can wiggle your fingers and toes and feel your feet on the floor and your fanny in the chair. Any and all of those things can help you settle down and refocus but *take your time*. This ain't the place for buckling down and forging ahead. In fact, as you'll see, dropping the rock-hard resilience posture is going to be key to healing from MTB.

MTB isn't something you can just press through. It requires a whole other set of skills to deal with. I'm talking soft skills like self-love, self-compassion, and patience. If you're just waking up to the fact that you've experienced medical trauma or have MTB, that's the first thing you need to process, by starting to understand and acknowledge what's happened *to* you, and what's now happening *inside* you.

I get it: All of this is a colossal shit-burger to be served by life. At the same time, it's a shit-burger that you don't have to eat. Rest assured that you *can* heal from MTB, and much of this book will discuss how.

So now that I've totally freaked you out, I'm also going to tell you don't worry. This is massive news and it's a lot to take in, but it is deal with-able. *Things can get better.* I am living proof of that.

One of the truly remarkable things about our brain-bodies is that we are always striving toward health. Even when it feels like we're far away, some part of us is always working to heal. Later in the book we're going to learn some approaches to support that part so it has some more resources to work with.

But for the moment, I want to just take a pause to acknowledge one particular emotion you might be feeling right about now. And in fact, it might be something you've actually been feeling for a while but haven't been aware of. That feeling is grief.

ACKNOWLEDGING GRIEF

We're going to talk more about grief and how to work with it in the second part of the book, but for now, I just want to make some space for all that you might be feeling in this moment, including grief. Grief is a complex emotion and experiencing it in this context—of chronic illness—is even more complex.

There's a lot of loss that comes with chronic illness. First, there's all the flat-out time you've spent being a patient, which can feel like years lost. Then there's the sadness of loss for things that can be hard to name, like the loss of the life you thought you'd have, the loss of your health, the loss of choices and options. The list goes on.

The whole thing can be hard to get your arms around. By comparison, if your pet dies, that's a known quantity. That's heartbreaking, but it's a kind of loss we're familiar with. We have a context for it. But with these other kinds of losses that aren't as easily defined, it can be harder to identify and, therefore, to identify our feelings about them. It can be difficult to feel justified in feeling grief or simply recognize that grief is part of what we're feeling. But here is the truth, dear friends: Grief is the loss of *anything* that matters to you.

Yet illness and the challenges associated with it are often ongoing, so closure simply isn't available, and that can make it difficult to "effectively" grieve. There's rarely a sense of, "Okay, that was tough, but I'm done with it now! I can move on." One of the reasons it's hard to get our arms around what we're feeling is that, well, it's difficult to get our arms around it. What I mean is, it's hard to come up with a cohesive narrative to describe what we've been through. And it's even tougher to explain those complexities to others. And because we don't have a language to describe or even understand what we're going through, it just goes unacknowledged. There's an element of vagueness or obscurity around our experiences, and that complicates our emotional process.

More good news, right? But try not to see this as a negative. Simply being able to identify that grief and loss are part of what you're feeling is a really powerful starting point. It's part of building back a foundation on which you can build going forward. But that's all to come. For now, baby steps.

Try to be kind with yourself as you process all of this. If you start to notice that you're having outsized reactions to things or just want to crawl under a rock, that's okay. I know that it feels terrible, but it will get better. You don't have to be the perfect patient or grieve-er or anything here. Just be you.

To support the healing journey, next we're going to get a deeper understanding of your body's stress-response system, along with a concept that pulls at the thread of MTB—something called *enduring somatic threat.* All of that will help us later when we start to gently loosen MTB's clammy yet surprisingly firm grip.

THREE

THE WILD RIDE OF FEAR LOOPING AND THE THREE *E*s

Alright team, are you ready to go back in? Because there's more to learn about trauma!

The worst pep talk ever, I know. It reminds me of a scene in the movie *Troop Beverly Hills*. Troop leader Shelley Long is standing there in front of her posh, polished gang of girls getting ready to lead them into the brambly snake-infested woods, and they're looking at her like, "Uh, you want us to go in *there*?" Yes, troop, we're going there.

Actually, I typically envision it more like a cave or a tunnel. The good news is that if you squint hard enough, you can see there's actually light at the other end. It's the light of freedom. But if I know only one thing, I know that the only way out is through.

I want to say here that you don't *have* to go back into the cave right now. As you work your way through this book, you'll start to see that a critical aspect of managing and recovering from trauma is learning to go at your own pace. Just like with chronic illness, you can't force or rush healing. Now's the time to start listening to yourself. To be (say it with me) *gentle.*

When my MTB was operating at full blast, nothing felt worse than not knowing what was "wrong" with me—why it seemed like I'd totally lost my marbles. But as much as it sucked, I wanted to be all up in this new info because I knew that's where the answers were. I am the type of person where, when I know I can do something to help myself, I lean all the way in. I was also aware that nothing could feel mentally worse than how I was feeling in that moment. So even though the future was daunting, I needed to get myself out of the cave.

Still, my journey of discovery unfolded over some time, whereas you're getting the whole kit and caboodle packaged up and dropped in your lap. Merry Christmas. What I had weeks and months to uncover and process, you're getting in hours, and that's a lot to work through. It might take a little time to let it all soak in and that's completely fine. The point is that it's your journey and it's your choice. As we go forward, you'll see that learning to trust yourself and your ability to know what's best for you is actually part of healing.

The thing with chronic illness is that (as we'll explore in detail in chapter 6) as patients we're often encouraged to let someone else make our decisions for us. After all, doctor knows best! It can be a massive shift in mindset to think of yourself as the captain of your own ship. Yet that's the role I'm inviting you to step into now. And it all starts with checking in with yourself to see how you're feeling and if you're ready for more.

There's also some really good news. The reason we're spending all this time unpacking trauma is that our brains and bodies are incredibly flexible. By flexible I mean changeable. Just like survival stress can turn to trauma, causing all kinds of things to rewire and recode inside us, that wiring and those codes can be changed. The process can be slow and, at times, pretty damn un-fun, but it's doable.

In the same way that our bodies are always trying to heal from illness, our brain-body is always up for healing from trauma. Again, that doesn't mean it's easy, but if you spark that energy of healing inside yourself, your brain-body will be all in with you, doing its very best to support you. Plus, I'll be here cheering, wearing my cap and face paint, pennant in one hand and big foam finger on the other, chanting, "You're number one!" until I'm hoarse.

But the fact remains: If at any point you need a breather, please take one. This book, and I, will be here (foam finger and all) when you're ready.

If the time to go on is now, then grab your safety gear and let's go! We're going to start by looking at one of my favorite (a term I'm using loosely here) concepts around trauma, which I call the Three Eeeks.

THE THREE *EEEKS*: EVENT, EXPERIENCE, EFFECTS

The Substance Abuse and Mental Health Services Administration (SAMHSA) came up with a model to help people understand and identify the impacts of trauma. They call it the Three *E*s, or as I like to call them the Three Eeeks . . . because *EEEK*!

According to SAMHSA, trauma is comprised of a potentially traumatic *Event*, the *Experience* of that event, and the long-term, lasting *Effects* of the event. Now, I use the phrase "potentially traumatic" because no event is inherently traumatic. Different people experience and process things differently. It's like the other day, Danny and I were in the car together, and suddenly, another car came out of nowhere and nearly hit us. Fortunately, Danny was able to slam on the breaks, stopping us in time to avoid an accident. Still, our stress responses had already been activated, dumping cortisol and other action-oriented hormones into our systems. Danny sat there wide-eyed for a few moments. "Holy shit, that was almost really bad," he said. But then he shook his head, took a deep breath, put the car back in gear, and went on with his day. Cut to me in the passenger seat and it was another story. I felt adrenaline rush through my body, my heart was pounding, and I felt frozen next to Danny in the car. I've found that's a pattern for me: After something stressful happens, I have to keep telling myself I'm safe long after everyone else is back to normal. I have to work significantly harder to calm myself down and do so intentionally. If I don't take extra measures to peel the icy fingers of trauma off me, I feel locked in a stress response. To be clear, I'm not saying the near miss was, by itself, *traumatic* for me. But this is a lingering effect of my MTB.

Survival stress doesn't always lead to lasting trauma. People can actually go through some pretty insane shit and not experience long-term negative effects. That doesn't mean those folks are stronger or better than someone who does experience trauma. That's kind of like saying blondes are better than redheads. It doesn't work that way. There are a ton of factors that contribute to how different experiences affect us—things like genes, personality, prior experiences, the culture we live in, and on and on. The point is simply that we're all different.

As SAMHSA describes it, "[T]rauma results from an event, series of events, or a set of circumstances that is experienced by an individual as physically [and/or] emotionally harmful, or life threatening, and that has lasting adverse effects on the individual's functioning and mental, physical, social, emotional, or spiritual well-being." Check, check, check, check, and check!

Let's look at an everyday instance where the Three *E*s could come into play. It's a lovely day and you're out for a walk. As you stroll along, you see a neighbor approaching with their dog. Everything seems fine and yet as you pass by, the pup suddenly lunges at you and bites your leg. Chaos erupts as your neighbor tries to get control of the dog, who's now barking at you, and you rush away. You're terrified and your leg is hurting. Suddenly you need to get some medical help, find out if the dog is current on his rabies shots, and so on.

Fortunately, the wound is minor and heals quickly. Still, now every time you see a dog approaching—even one who seems friendly—you tense up and your heart starts racing. You cross the street to get away from the dog or, if that's not possible, give it as wide a berth as you can. It's sad because you always liked dogs in the past, but now when you see them, you're worried they'll go Cujo on you.

In this case, the event would have been the dog lunging and biting. The experience would have included the sights, sounds, smells, and abject terror (the feels) of having a pleasant situation when your guard was totally down shift so suddenly into one where you feared for your safety and health. And the effect was the newfound fear of dogs that continued long after your physical wounds had healed.

Now that you've got the gist, let's shift gears to look at some of the trauma that caused my MTB through the lens of the Three *E*s:

- **Event:** Me getting sick (again!). When I was exposed to the hideous black mold in my apartment and learned that my own home was unsafe and making me sick.
- **Experience:** The sights, sounds, smells, and feelings when I got sick. I became highly allergic to, like, *everything*, and became

physically hyperreactive not only to mold but also to chemicals like the kind in household cleaners and the scents added to (as I discovered) virtually every product under the sun.

- **Effects:** I was handed an express ticket to the hell between sick and well. In addition to the physical effects, I experienced lasting mental effects. Because I was allergic to so many environmental factors, I was so worried about having to protect myself from having a reaction that I'd often be uncomfortable in any new place. I'd stress out, sometimes to the point of a panic attack. It was as if some part of me thought that my anxiety or forward-planning would somehow insulate me from the event actually happening. I went in hypervigilance as a means of protecting myself. I obsessed and prepared for the worst. It was like I didn't have a problem-solving gear. I didn't trust myself to troubleshoot if I started noticing any issues—either with my physical or my mental health. Because I was so caught off guard by the toxic exposure, my irrational mind thought that I would need to be aware and alert constantly to it happening again. It was like I was a glass of a seltzer that had bubbled to the top, and it became my "job" to make sure it didn't overflow because that would just be TOO MUCH.

When things go haywire inside us like this, it's because of changes in our stress response system. Remember in chapter 2 how Dr. Robert Scaer described how with trauma, something goes wonky with our procedural memory? Something can trigger our brain-body into "responding to internal cues of a threat that no longer exists." Suddenly we're reacting to something in our past rather than what's actually happening in the here and now. We get into a *fear loop*. But unlike a Froot Loop, this loop is neither fun nor delicious.

STUCK IN THE FEAR LOOP

Have you ever had that experience where you wake up in the middle of the night to the incessant chirping of a smoke alarm? (Why on God's green earth do the batteries in those things always seem to die at 3 a.m.?) You wake up startled, your mind awash with confusion. Before you gain clarity and realize what's happening, all you know is that something's wrong, and your brain is searching frantically to figure out what it is. That's what it's like to be triggered into a fear loop. All the screens flash on in your brain as it starts scanning your body trying to determine where the threat is. In the meantime, you're on high alert. Heart racing, hands shaking . . . Or for others, the alarm can trigger more of a shutdown or dissociative response, where perhaps you start to get fuzzy and numb out. Maybe you go into a type of freeze mode where you feel like you can't take any action at all. You're just sitting there staring at the thing like, "Huh?"

Let's take the fire alarm metaphor one step further. The next time you're sleeping and you hear so much as a single chirp from one of those things, or any sound that is chirp-adjacent, you bolt upright in bed, listening with all your might, straining to hear whether the chirp will become an onslaught of steady beeping. That's what hypervigilance is like. We go into self-protective mode—a space that's supposed to be temporary—and never come out. Now you're in the fear loop.

Here's what's important to understand about this scenario: Our initial bolt-up-in-bed, "Dear God, what's happening?!" response is a natural reaction to the sudden, unknown stressor of the alarm. When we first hear the noise, we don't know what the heck's happening, so our body automatically goes into protective mode and floods with survival stress (and all the chemicals that go with it). You've likely heard the trauma metaphor involving the tiger. If a tiger leaps out at you, the fear you feel is a normal and healthy response because it's designed to save your ass. That's why it's called survival stress. It ensures that your attention is directed on the threat—the tiger. The fear, by itself, is not a trauma response. As long as we can shake it off, this incident does not lead to lasting trauma. It's when we can't shake it off—meaning process it out—that we have a problem. That's you launching into fear every time something prompts a memory (whether conscious or not) of the incident. That's you avoiding the spot where the tiger leapt at you. That's you bolting upright in bed hearing something that faintly resembles a chirping sound. That's what can lead to fear looping, and *that's* a trauma response (we'll go into more detail about our responses to survival stress in the next chapter). When we have trauma, we sometimes have trouble distinguishing what's a threat and what's not.

Trauma expert Peter Levine explains in his book *Waking the Tiger* that the reason an antelope won't develop trauma after an unsuccessful tiger attack is that it will literally shake (and shiver) off the incident, then go on with its life. That's how the animal processes out the stress and *completes* it. But humans tend not to be quite so good at shaking things off.

Remember how I explained in the last chapter that people with chronic illness often hold on to survival stress and don't know *how* to go back and process it out? All that survival stress gets stored inside us and leads to fear loops.

THE WORLD'S WORST TRAIN RIDE: THE PHASES OF THE FEAR LOOP

Here's a six-phase model that maps out the stops along the fear loop. There are actually multiple models out there and each is slightly different. Some also call it a *trauma loop*. This is my own greatest hits mash-up version.

1. **Activation Town:** Something happens that activates the response. This is the whole distorted memory idea where something that's not directly related to the original event triggers us into survival mode.
2. **Conditioned Response-ville:** The automatic response kicks in. This can look like fear, anxiety, panic, or it can be more like numbing or checking out. It can also include physical symptoms like your heart pounding in your chest or losing feeling in your extremities.
3. **Avoidance Acres:** You try to avoid anything that might trigger you.
4. **Hypervigilance Hills:** In order to try to identify any potential trigger source, you become more vigilant than the president's Secret Service detail.
5. **Repetition Circle:** Play it back! This is the looping part. This cycle happens over, and over, and over again, each time getting more and more deeply embedded into your circuitry. Cue the hamster wheel.
6. **Constricted Reality Boulevard:** You start to see the world through the narrow lens of potential triggers that you're trying to avoid. From this perspective, life starts to feel small and threatening. This is where our baseline changes as we start to get used to the state and the feeling of our nervous system being flooded. Overwhelm becomes the norm.

As you can see, the fear loop isn't just a nice little scenic flat loop on a kiddie train, it's a downward spiral to a fresh hell. I wish I was exaggerating, but that's really what it feels like when it's happening. But if you're anything like me, you already know that.

Dr. Bruce Perry, a renowned trauma expert, describes what's going on in our brain when we're in this loop despite the fact that the original threat is no longer there. A key part, he says, is that you're in a state of unrelenting perpetual fear. (Sounds nice, right?) In *What Happened to You?* (a book he co-wrote with Oprah), he writes, "A person will think, learn, feel, and behave differently when they are afraid compared to when they feel safe.... All functioning of the brain is 'state-dependent.' At any given moment, the collective status of our body's systems and the mind's attention determines the state we're in—and our state can change very quickly."

You see, a healthy brain has varying states of arousal. You can think of general arousal as a kind of alertness. Throughout a given day, it's normal for you to cycle through various states of being more relaxed or being more awake and attentive.

When we're calm, we have access to the "smartest" part of our brain (meaning it has the highest level of control over our thoughts and actions)—that's the prefrontal cortex. When we're relaxed, the prefrontal cortex is online and our mind can wander and drift.

When we suddenly shift into a hyper-alert or hyper-aroused state, we're in alarm mode, and that alarm essentially drowns out our prefrontal cortex. So, while the PFC wants to inject some calm and rationality up in here, we can't hear it. Instead, we're racing around, hands flapping, shrieking for help. In other words, we lose control of our emotions and they start running the show.

Dr. Perry explains that in this state, our problem-solving skills can deteriorate and we can become laser focused on the present. We lose our ability to pan back and inject some perspective into the situation (That's not an actual tiger; it's just a box of Frosted Flakes!). When you're in this mode, there is no spaciousness, *you are all up in it.* As you can imagine, getting stuck in that state is not a great place to be. When I get triggered I lose the ability to self-regulate. It feels like there is no amount of self-soothing or deep breathing in the world that can calm me down. I rocket so quickly into fight-or-flight mode that I experience a physical-emotional time warp that makes it almost impossible for me to be in the present moment. It's like in an instant, I'm right back in the struggle for survival.

When I spoke to nervous system expert Irene Lyon, she said that when our nervous system is super dysregulated, we often try to manage that discomfort by controlling things. That can look like overriding your body's impulses, like needing to have a snack, go to bed, or trying to have rigid control over your surroundings or your routine. For me, it presented like a kind of obsessive-compulsive thinking where I felt like I needed to be so hypervigilant about my surroundings in order to keep myself safe.

As Lyon described it when we spoke, "It shows that we have a very thin window of tolerance or we have no window of tolerance. If we have no window of tolerance, we are not regulated." She continued, "Most people in the West have a fake window of tolerance. So, they push and they override, they live in what we call a *functional freeze* state. And what often occurs is they crash. There's an event that happens. I've seen this with people getting into car accidents, there'll be a death in the family, a natural disaster, and they'll get derailed." But unlike someone with a regulated nervous system, the event knocks them totally off-kilter and they can't find their footing again. Instead, they spiral.

For me, I thought I was better in every way, and then I got mold poisoning, and I unraveled. This new dimension of sickness, in addition to the global pandemic, sent my stress levels over the edge. As Lyon explained to me, my thread was thin.

I shared what getting triggered looks like for me, but here are some other ways it can manifest. One of my clients has been cancer free for seven full years but still gets nauseated when they simply read or hear the word "chemotherapy." One doctor I work with told me about a patient who had emergency heart surgery years before but still suffers panic attacks, sometimes to the point of dissociation, when they have to get a routine physical. Another client of mine used to get palsy-like symptoms every day for years that she thought were caused by hemiplegic migraines. Later she found out that she had a tick-borne infection. While that infection has long since healed and she no longer has either headaches or paralysis in her face, any time she feels anything that could remotely signal the onset of a headache, she goes into total panic, convinced that her face will freeze again.

It's like me when I get anywhere near grass. Yes, grass. Something that feels so welcoming and enjoyable and grounding to others sends me fear looping. Since my Lyme diagnosis, when I'm in grass I worry obsessively about ticks. The mindfuck of it is that we actually *do* need to be aware and vigilant about these little blood suckers, and to a certain extent it's totally rational to be vigilant. (Plus, we are totally not equipped to prevent this growing disease in our country!) But whereas others can simply do the comb and shake routine after some time in the cool, lush grass, simply checking for ticks and being done with it, my tick-phobia takes over. Or at least, it used to.

Last year after a trip to the farmers market, I was holding a nice bunch of greens and, I kid you not, a tick hopped right off them and onto my shirt where it proceeded to make a beeline (a tick line?) for my exposed skin! My stress response kicked in like a mofo. Right away I trapped and killed the little fucker and guess what? A major panic attack *did not* ensue. I assured myself I was safe, and it was over, and I trusted my ability to handle it if there was an actual problem. It felt like a miracle. And get this: A few months before that, Danny and I were at the beach, and I walked by a cluster of beach grass *right through the sand with my bare feet* and didn't freak out! I didn't realize I was walking on grass anymore. The monumental nature of that was not lost on Danny. "Look what you just did!" he cheered. So while I'm still working my way off the terror train (baby steps!), for me the fear loop is no longer a given. And that's what I'm hoping you take from this—the awareness that while right now you might be on the world's worst train ride, it doesn't always have to be like this. In time you can get off. You will have the power to get off the train, wait at the station, and take an Acela of your choosing.

I also want to assure you that this shit is real. Meaning, it's not just all in your head. As Dr. Scaer writes: "There is nothing 'inappropriate' or 'psychological' about these responses, for they are precipitated by new pathways in brain centers that remain devoted to the endless task of escaping from the old, unresolved threat." In other words, you're not just being a crazy, hysterical mess when this happens—someone who should just get your shit together (or take a Xanax!). The fear loop is the result of *actual changes* that have happened inside you.

Now that we get the idea of the Three *E*s and fear loops, let's take a big breath, then go one step deeper in understanding MTB.

It's time to talk about post-traumatic stress disorder and its newly identified sister from another mister, complex post-traumatic stress disorder (you know, for those times when regular old PTSD just doesn't feel like enough). And to get there we're going to start with yet another acronym: EST.

ENDURING SOMATIC THREAT

When I dove into the topic of trauma on a quest to find out more about how it affects people with chronic illness, I went deep. I spent hours online, downloaded scientific papers, watched documentaries, and you should see the stacks of books in my apartment.

Along the way I came across a researcher named Dr. Donald Edmondson, a professor in the Department of Psychiatry at Columbia University. In his work, Edmondson actually landed on a term that described some of the way I'd been feeling. In 2015, Edmondson published a paper on post-traumatic stress in acute life-threatening medical events, things like getting into a bad car accident or having a stroke or heart attack. As a practicing neurologist, he was seeing a lot of these patients in his own practice. Edmondson found that such experiences can have lingering mental and emotional effects. Check out this comment he quoted in his paper, which comes from a response to a 2012 *New York Times* article on PTSD in heart attack survivors:

> *"I have never been the same since. I suffer from extreme anxiety, hyper vigilance and a host of other psychological symptoms related to my cardiac history. I am hyper aware of every extra or missed heart beat, which brings me right back to the original arrhythmia. I struggle on a daily basis to do the most basic things."*

Sound familiar?

As Edmondson explains, people have long recognized that we can develop PTSD as the result of an acute life-threatening event. (For reference, Dr. Bruce Perry describes PTSD in terms of the Three *E* model, saying, "PTSD is about the effects." Specifically, it's a "cluster of symptoms" that can "occur in the wake of a traumatic event or events.")

In Edmondson's view, there are significant and important differences between the kind of PTSD a patient experiences from a single traumatic event, like a stroke, and "ongoing medical illness." He writes: "[T]he re-experiencing symptoms of PTSD due to a medical illness are often focused on enduring threats of recurrence and functional decline rather than on a discrete event in the past whose danger has passed." In other words, EST ain't your mama's PTSD.

Classically, PTSD has been associated with a single event (or potentially multiple events over a short period of time) that induced massive survival stress. But when you have a chronic illness, the event occurs over a long period of time, over and over again, because the event isn't actually going away. Your body *is* the event.

Essentially, you're carrying the scene of your trauma around with you because it *is* you. That means you're more likely to get triggered. The trigger—the cue that sends your nervous system into flooding and overwhelm—could be outside you, like the smell of hospital antiseptic or the hum of an MRI machine. Or it could be inside, like the halo that foreshadows a migraine or the body aches that signal systemic inflammation. These sensations can lead to feelings and behaviors such as anxiety, avoidance, and heightened emotional responses.

My friend spent years doing a nasty dance with colitis. Through it all, there were tests and surgeries and appointment after appointment. Fortunately, she's doing way better now and hasn't had any major symptoms in years. However, she recently noticed something. Every time she gets on a table—whether it's at the doctor's office for her routine physical, at the acupuncturist's office, or snuggling down for a massage—something inside her shifts. It's like she kind of zones out, but not in the relaxed way. Some part of her *goes away.* When she talked to another friend who's trauma-literate, the friend said, "Dude, you're dissociating."

It's another version of the fear loop. Instead of her getting all worked up with a certain set of cues—like being a patient on a table—she actually numbs out. When she explored this idea further, she realized it happens at other times, too, like when she has to make a high-stakes decision about something. She goes into a kind of freeze state where she feels unable to take action. I, as you've probably guessed, have the opposite reaction. I go into extreme hypervigilance and become almost *too* present to what's happening. Yet I also tend to experience a paralysis around decision making. That just illustrates the big range in how different people can respond to survival stress and trauma.

In my reading, I discovered that the phenomenon that I call Medical Trauma Brain might—at least for some people—fall under a newer diagnosis: *complex* post-traumatic stress disorder, or CPTSD.

While mental health docs aren't yet all on the same page about exactly what constitutes CPTSD versus PTSD, they do agree on one thing. It's that PTSD is more defined by a single or short-term experience of intense survival stress, whereas the territory of CPTSD is continuous trauma over a longer period of time. Think: a single instance of assault versus years of abuse. Sounds like long-term chronic illness, no?

When it comes to diagnostic criteria, psychologists tend to describe CPTSD as the touring edition of your favorite SUV. It's got all of the features of PTSD *and more*! Specifically, the CPTSD package adds on something called a disturbance in self-organization (DSO).

I don't know about you, but I'm extremely well organized. Unfortunately, that's not what DSO is about. It means that the affected person may experience difficulties with affect regulation, self-concept, or relationships. In the language normal people speak, affect regulation means the ability to regulate your emotions. Issues with self-concept could look like feelings of being worthless or ongoing guilt, or a fragmented sense of self where you feel like you're essentially bad or broken in some way. It could be difficult to maintain a stable sense of who you are and how you walk through the world, which, not surprisingly, can negatively affect your ability to manage your emotions and maintain healthy relationships. Remember how I said it was like I had lost my baseline? Feeling baseless or disoriented can actually be a symptom of MTB.

Okay, let's hit the pause button. That last part was super in the weeds, I know (I warned you we were going into the woods!). There's a whole lot more out there on PTSD and CPTSD if you want to read about them in more detail. For now, I wanted to share enough to familiarize you with them in the context of MTB.

But guess what? You made it! We're not all the way through the cave yet, but we're nearly there. In the next chapter we're going to go into a little more detail about the various ways our nervous system can respond to survival stress, and how MTB can look.

Now stand up and shake it out. When you're ready, we'll embark on a more in-depth look at your survival system—how it helps you, and how it can go haywire.

FOUR

ALL THE EFFING *F*s

Welcome back! I'm glad you're sticking with me. And I also hope you're taking those breaks—doing those meditations, taking baths, downing wheatgrass shots, jamming to reggae . . . basically whatever supports you any time you feel maxed out. Take that as my prescription for you: one dose of whatever makes you feel better (that's not totally unhealthy), as needed. Because make no mistake about it, this is some tough shit. That's just a fact. But here's another fact: So are you. *You can do this!* And I (and Super Freak) got your back.

That said, let's journey back into the cave! In today's episode of *What the Fucking Fuck?!* we're taking a look at some of the specific ways our nervous system can respond to trauma. Specifically, we're unpacking all the Effing *F*s, as I so fondly call them: *fight, flight, freeze, flock,* and *fawn.* The reason we're going there is that understanding these responses will help you recognize and track them and eventually be able to re-route them so they don't take over your psyche and rocket you off into oblivion.

At its height, my response to MTB included frequent anxiety attacks coupled with extreme episodes of fear, to the point that even the *idea* of a threat to my health made me feel unsafe in the world, my home, even my own skin. I grew inflexible and rigid almost to the point of compulsion because I lived in a state of ghastly, unrelenting, perpetual dread. It became impossible to distinguish between what was uncomfortable and what was dangerous. On top of this burning pile of shit, it was hard to trust myself because even the most well-intentioned health care professionals and loved ones either downplayed and ignored my instincts, or fully gaslit me for so long, making me feel like I was going crazy. I don't blame them—they all wanted me to be better—but it was a perfect recipe for trauma.

While I was working on this book, I had the honor of speaking with Dr. Gabor Maté. I asked him to describe how he views trauma, and I absolutely loved what he said because I resonated with it so strongly. He said, "Trauma is not what happened to you as a child, but it is what happened inside you as a result of what happened to you. Trauma literally means a wound—that's the meaning of the word. A wound is not in the past. It's in the present. It's an unhealed wound. So if you sustained a blow to the head two years ago and you still had post-concussion syndrome, that's the wound. So trauma is what you're carrying inside in the present as a result of what happened way back. It's an unhealed psychological wound."

In *The Myth of Normal*, Dr. Maté writes, "[T]rauma is a psychic injury, lodged in our nervous system, mind, and body, lasting long past the originating incident(s), triggerable at any moment. It is a constellation of hardships, composed of the wound itself and the residual burdens that our woundedness imposes on our bodies and souls." *Residual burdens.* It so perfectly captures the experience of MTB. It's like a ghost in the house.

And the thing is, even though trauma is a psychic wound, that doesn't mean it only affects the psyche. As Dr. Maté explained when we spoke, "Mind and body can't be separated. It's all one unit. There's no such thing as isolated psychic wounds that don't have psychological implications. And the emotional system and the immune system are, for example, one unit, they're not separate systems."

When I spoke with Irene Lyon, she echoed this idea, saying, "Trauma is not in the brain, it's not in the thinking, it's not even in the behavior. It's in the autonomic nervous system. Survival physiology, and all of the branches of it, how we connect, how we connect to the environment, how we mount a threat response, how we come out of a threat response, how our organ systems work, our immune system, endocrine, cardiovascular respiratory . . . all the things."

That's why trauma in general, and for our purposes MTB in particular, affects us so deeply and so broadly. And that's what we're unpacking here.

In previous chapters we talked about survival stress. Now we're going to look at the responses that stress can trigger inside us.

CHOOSE YOUR *F*

You're probably already somewhat familiar with the idea of fight-flight-freeze as that space our brain-bodies go to when we sense a potentially serious threat. When something prompts our insides to sound the alarm, our brain-bodies automatically prepare us for a response. We might move toward the threat (fight), try to move away from it (flight), or seize up (freeze). Many different factors can influence our response, like what the actual threat is, our personality, our previous life experiences, and so on. You might freeze when you're in a situation where neither fight nor flight is an option.

Fight, flight, and freeze are automatic, physiological responses to acute survival stress. So in the moment that stress spikes—whether it's because an actual tiger jumps out at you or it's just a friend yelling "Surprise!" and startling the you-know-what out of you—it causes a reaction inside you. In the moment you sense a threat, on a fundamental level your nervous system reacts. And it's a good thing it does. As Irene Lyon describes them, the fight, flight, and freeze responses are "survival strategies that we humans use to stay safe when we are in the midst of scary things that are happening to us." In other words, these survival strategies are valuable tools that we need to get through life.

To get a sense of what they're all about, let's look at these modes in action. Say you're out at a bar with some friends and you accidentally spill your drink on the drunk stranger next to you. Drunkie gets all belligerent and wants to start something. The situation escalates quickly as he starts screaming in your face. Sensing danger, your body floods with survival stress. In that moment you don't know if this dude is just being a *jerk* or whether he could become seriously unhinged. As a result, your whole physiology shifts you into automatic response mode.

Now, we often have a go-to response—we're either a fighter, a flight-er, or a freezer. But we can also shift among them depending on the situation and how it unfolds. Back at the bar, your knee-jerk response may be to want to throw down (fight). "Bring it on, sucka!" Or, you might be more inclined to toss a twenty on the bar and start hustling your gal pals toward the door (flight). That's me! Or you might go into bug-eyed mode where your mouth clamps shut, your joints lock, and you're unsure what to do (freeze). You know how in period movies when something shocking happens, some woman will inevitably gasp, clutch her pearls, and then drop to the floor? Going lights out is actually an extreme freeze response.

Now, in case all of this didn't seem fun enough, there are two other potential responses that psychologists have begun to talk about, which are *flock* and *fawn*. (And some describe even more *F*s, but I think these two are both more widely accepted at this point and more relevant to MTB.) The difference with these two *F*s is that, unlike fight, flight, and freeze, they aren't just automatic responses generated by our nervous system. You can think of them more like *social strategies* that we can use to keep us safe.

Flocking is about looking to see how others in your group are responding, or how they're encouraging you to respond. In the example of our drunkie at the bar, you might look to your friends to see what *they* think you should do—whether they're urging you to take a swing or GTF out of Dodge.

Another option is to apologize to the drunk. That's considered fawning behavior, where we try to appease the source of the threat. But instead of offering just an "I'm so sorry I spilled my drink on you," you're all, "I'm so clutzy, please forgive me, I'll pay for your drink, no I'll pay for your whole tab!" Fawning is about trying to avoid conflict by putting aside your own feelings or needs to placate someone else. You're trying to manage them to dial down the intensity of the situation. Not-so-fun fact: That's why they say that people-pleasing behavior can be a trauma response.

But here's something that's important to understand: All of these *F*s are potentially normal, healthy responses to survival stress. None of them is necessarily a *trauma* response. For instance, a healthy fight response can either help you take on a literal threat to your safety, or it can help you stand up for yourself.

Psychotherapist Pete Walker does a nice job describing some of the positive aspects of our *F* responses. He writes in a blog post:

> *"Easy access to the fight response insures good boundaries, healthy assertiveness and aggressive self-protectiveness if necessary. Untraumatized individuals also easily and appropriately access their flight instinct and disengage and retreat when confrontation would exacerbate their danger. They also*

> *freeze appropriately and give up and quit struggling when further activity or resistance is futile or counterproductive. And finally they also fawn in a liquid, 'play-space' manner and are able to listen, help, and compromise as readily as they assert and express themselves and their needs, rights and points of view."*

This is what happens when you have a *regulated nervous system* and can move in and out of this survival mode relatively easily. For kicks, let's say a tiger does jump out at you and immediately your stress level goes to eleven. Then, you see that it's not actually a tiger, it's just your neighbor's docile greyhound dressed in a tiger costume for Halloween. With a healthy nervous system, you can sigh, laugh, and go back to normal.

It's like when Danny and I almost got in a car accident and he was able to shake it off and go on with his day. Not so for me, who was shaking and quaking for the next few hours. That's because my nervous system? It ain't so regulated.

Picture a horizontal line. On one end is chill space (low arousal), and on the other is alert space (high arousal). When our nervous system is regulated, we can easily slide back and forth on this spectrum depending on what's going on. But when it's *dysregulated*, a few things can happen. For one, we can get stuck in the high arousal zone (where fight and flight live) and have a hard time getting out of it. Or if we're in the low arousal zone, the slightest thing can send us rocketing to the other side. We can also get stuck in the low arousal zone. That's where the freeze response lives. The point is we don't move back and forth easily or smoothly.

Trauma and a dysregulated nervous system go together like peanut butter and jelly. For those of us with MTB, our janky nervous systems can make our stress response go haywire in all the ways I mentioned above. On top of that our triggers can get mis-wired. So something that's totally separate from the original scary incident can send us into survival mode. I know someone who gets the shakes every time she smells Lysol because it reminds her of the hospital. That's a dysfunctional response because there's no actual threat in the moment—her brain-body just *thinks* there is.

As I mentioned a moment ago, anyone can engage any of the *F*s depending on the situation. Generally I go into survival mode and engage the *F*s when I feel like I have to defend myself, or when I feel like something has to be done a certain way to keep me safe and someone else disagrees or isn't taking the threat to my health seriously. (And it's an actual threat—not just me being dysregulated.) For example, if we're traveling I'll reach out to the place we're staying and ask that scent-free and hypoallergenic products be used so I don't have an allergic reaction. Before, I used to *completely* stress out about whether they'd do that or not, but now I just ask and know that if they don't, I'll figure it out. (And yes, I'm aware that request might come across to some as high maintenance, but I'm voicing it because chemical sensitivities are *way* more common than many people realize. Just ask someone who's been through chemo.)

Hypervigilance and catastrophizing are some other greatest hits for me. When I get totally overwhelmed by a situation, I get analysis paralysis and cannot make a decision to save my life. All of a sudden, my brain lights up like a supercomputer, simultaneously calculating eighty-thousand distinct possibilities. It becomes too much to think about and my brain just fogs over.

Flock and Fawn are also good friends of mine. When I feel overwhelmed, I throw myself at the feet of the doctor, the teacher, the healer, the coach, looking to them for answers to my ordeal based on their superior all-knowingness.

Then there's my all-time MTB BFF: fawning. In my health journey, this has happened *a lot*, where I apologize for being "too much." My fawning mode auto-engages every time I get a short response from a doctor, or an off glance or opinion from a loved one. I feel the need to apologize to make sure the dynamic—especially with the doctor—remains safe and everyone feels good about it. I make sure that everyone feels important and valued, EVEN if the narrative has me doubting my own experiences. Speaking of *F*s, how fucked is THAT?

So, there you go—my rogues' gallery of survival stress responses, any of which can get activated when I'm fear looping. It's a really wild ride. But let's look at some other examples.

Remember the friend mentioned in the last chapter who tends to numb out when she's on any kind of treatment table? That kind of shutting down and going inside yourself (which, again, is technically called *dissociation*) is one type of freeze response.

When I was working on this chapter, I spoke to my friend Simon, who has been struggling with long COVID and a host of related health challenges. When I described to him the idea of MTB and the feeling of The Shadowlands, he knew exactly what I was talking about. For him it feels like a place that is dark, where he can't feel the ground beneath him. He calls crashing into that bottomless spiral The Dumps. When he's there, it's hard for him to even describe what he's feeling, he is so overwhelmed and inundated, so he came up with this shorthand to help his wife understand where he is.

As it happened, he suffered a terrible bout of The Dumps two nights before we spoke. One of the spinoffs of Simon's long COVID is mast cell activation syndrome (MCAS), which makes him *extremely* sensitive to histamine. That day, while other New Yorkers had been out frolicking in the happy sunshine of early spring,

Simon's antennae were already up due to the extreme amount of pollen in the air. He'd been wearing his mask all day to be preventative. Regardless of his protective strategy, the counts were so high that he'd had some serious exposure. It was enough to send Simon into The Dumps (a.k.a. The Shadowlands). But he didn't just feel bad physically. When his tripwire was triggered, as he told me, he was also overcome by these massive waves of *anger*, at everyone and everything. Even his totally innocent and completely loving wife. That night as he was taking a shower he felt flooded with the urge to start a fight—it didn't matter who with.

This is the part that struck me. Simon said that when he's in The Dumps, it's like he's getting hijacked—like there's this shadow in the room that just takes over every part of him. Suddenly he's in this place where he's not perceiving reality correctly. In the snap of a finger he can go from being okay to feeling like the whole world is against him.

It turns out that Simon's survival stress response is a pretty solid fighter. And because it's a trauma response, it can go way overboard. One time he described for me how several years into suffering severely from long COVID, if a food delivery person came to the door and wasn't wearing a mask, he'd absolutely lose his shit on them, accusing them of trying to kill him and his wife by potentially exposing them to COVID. After all, he knew all-too-well the horrors that COVID can unleash. Then he'd call Uber and complain, *loudly*. He would totally come apart and spend all this time and energy seeking justice. As time went on, Simon noticed that just the sound of someone at the door—whether it was a delivery driver or an unexpected knock—would send him into panic mode. His mind would shoot directly to his worst-case scenario: that the delivery person would have no mask on and he would once again be exposed to COVID. His heart would accelerate as his body filled with extreme fear. All of this was because he was afraid of getting sick all over again.

We'll talk about Simon more in the second part of the book, but for now, I'll say that while he's still struggling with The Dumps and fear looping, today he's much more aware, and his reactions aren't so automatic and unbridled. Like me, he's learning to invoke strategies that can help to turn down the volume on his trauma response.

As you let all of that sink in, now might be a good time to take a pause and reflect on some of your own experiences. Do you tend to have a default mode? If so, what is it? What are times you can recall engaging some of the other modes? What does that look and feel like?

This isn't a one-and-done reflection. As you move toward healing, you'll start to more easily recognize where and how you've embodied these responses in the past, and you'll also start to be able to identify when they're flaring up in real time. Recognition and awareness are the first step to recovery. That's a good thing because it's an essential step to defusing some of these reactions and shifting gears in situations when they're not actually helpful. Because that's what happens with MTB, when our stress response goes haywire and we start fear looping.

Now, there's another mode I came across when researching trauma that I think is extremely helpful to understanding the experience of MTB. It's something called *functional freeze,* and when I describe what it is, I have a feeling you're gonna have an "Oh shit!" moment, just like I did when I learned about it.

THE OTHER *F*: FUNCTIONAL FREEZE

Okay, so technically *functional freeze* has two *F*s but you know what I mean. And honestly, it feels like a double *F*. Unlike the other *F*s, functional freeze isn't just an immediate response to survival stress. Instead, it's ongoing, like a really shitty state of being.

With functional freeze, some part of us is essentially in a kind of shut-down state—the freeze mode. Only we're not totally frozen, we're still doing stuff. Especially in our culture, we tend not to be very good at caring for ourselves (have ya noticed?). We don't stay home and rest when we've got a cold, we don't slow down when we're tired, and we don't give ourselves the time and space to heal from mental and emotional wounds. I get it—kids gotta go to soccer, bills gotta get paid—but an unfortunate downside is that even when our brain-bodies are telling us, "I need help!" we press on. It's that damn toxic resilience again. And we never circle back to resolve or process the original issue, feelings, etc.

My friend Kira shared some of her experience with this. She was diagnosed with rheumatoid arthritis when she was sixteen. She's now a mom of two, working in one of those corporate jobs that feels soul-sucking, but she feels trapped because it offers good insurance that pays for her $4,000-per-month injections. It's the golden handcuffs. Without the insurance she'd have to go back on a lower-cost medication that doesn't work as well and makes her feel terrible. It's a hideous choice: Get the care you need but be stuck in a job you hate or leave and be cast out into health care no-man's-land.

Then there's just the day-to-day of balancing a full-time job with a chronic illness. Kira said that for her, The Shadowlands feels less like a desert wasteland and more like a giant crush, like she's getting squeezed between two walls. One wall is the demands of her illness and managing her symptoms, and the other is the demands of work and the expectation that you show up and perform. When she has to take a sick day, she worries that people see her as somehow morally weak, like her RA is somehow a personal failing. She feels like if she's not "sick enough," she has to just push through and keep working—that she can't justify taking time to rest so she doesn't feel even worse. As she told me, "It's like I'll be here working or be off and don't exist. There's no in-between." Oh, and add to it the responsibilities of being a wife and mother. Those added demands, along with work and RA, are all just impossible to manage simultaneously. You literally cannot do it all. And that ongoing stress adds to the mental-emotional burden that people with chronic illness are already carrying.

The pressures Kira feels are both external and internal. "It often manifests as guilt," she told me. "I'm never doing enough, especially as a working mother. It feels like it's never enough in any sphere and there isn't really any help for that. I feel this general dis-ease, or unease, a lot of the time. It's like, you aren't really up to it, but you have to show up anyway. The deficit between those two things can be a fence of self-criticality, like guilt, or low-grade depression. It's this sense of thirst or depletion, like you never quite have what you need." Once again, toxic resilience culture rears its ugly head!

The fact that we still do stuff in spite of the fact that some part of us is in overwhelm or shut-down mode is why they call it *functional* freeze. Irene Lyon has a useful way to describe it, like driving your car with the brake on. If you picture that you are the car, imagine what it feels like to simultaneously have your brakes on and also have the pedal to the metal. There are warring chemicals and emotions doing battle inside you, with one side wanting you to slow down and the other urging you to keep going.

Not surprisingly, spending a lot of time in this state (I'm talking months, years, decades . . . even a lifetime) eventually causes the system to break down, just like a car would. Imagine how much energy you expend trying to keep these two modes going all the time. Lyon explains that living in functional freeze mode can be so taxing that it can lead to a variety of chronic syndromes. And that's one of the ways that long-term trauma can lead to physical illness. (Something you don't need any more of, thank you very much.)

Functional freeze can lead to mental and emotional challenges as well. For instance, it can make you feel demotivated, disconnected, or depressed, or it can shift you into shut-down mode when you become overwhelmed and your nervous system becomes flooded. That's the space where just ONE MORE THING is enough to tip the scales, and it doesn't really matter what it is. You could be standing at the grocery store looking for your favorite hummus and *it's not friggin there! What the hell is wrong with these people? Can't you just get some damn hummus around here already?! WHY IS LIFE SO HARD?!* [Cut to you standing there sobbing in the Dips and Spreads section or going off on the stock person.]

Or maybe instead of freaking out you go into total shut-down mode, balling up on your couch and disengaging. Or, first one, then the other. It can look different ways for different people, or at different times.

It's important to note that Lyon says that one of the reasons we get into this mode and stay trapped there is because at some point in our lives, we had an experience where we needed to *process* survival stress and couldn't. We couldn't let the stress *complete*. We couldn't express our feelings or emotions. Instead, our response was stopped. It was cut off, either by ourselves or someone else or by the circumstances. That can predispose us to going into freeze mode later in life. In any event, I bet you can connect some dots here. All of those experiences where you leaned on resilience and never expressed those emotions or processed those feelings about your chronic illness may have landed you a functional freeze. Or it could be due to other experiences in your life and MTB compounded it. Either way, I see functional freeze as a common aspect of MTB, and so it's useful to understand. I have spent a lot of time in those frozen waters in the middle of the lake with no paddle. It is a very lonely place to be.

In his book *Power Healing* my own doctor, Leo Galland, describes an experience with a patient who he calls Miguel. Dr. Galland met Miguel when he arrived at the hospital basically on the brink of death. Fortunately, Dr. Galland and his team were able to resolve Miguel's mystery illness, but that wasn't the end of Miguel's story.

Dr. Galland writes: "Three months later, I sat talking to Miguel in the outpatient clinic. He was a nervous wreck; he couldn't sleep; he was losing time from his job and had lost all desire for sex with his wife. The reason was no mystery. He was afraid the sickness would return. Twice in five years he had almost died. Why should he believe it wouldn't happen again?"

Some part of Miguel was stuck in the fear loop. He was trying to move on but he struggled to engage with his life again. Something inside him had changed. He was attempting to function, but he was in perpetual overwhelm.

There's another image Irene Lyon invokes that I think is really helpful here when it comes to why we can get so overwhelmed at times. Why something can happen that suddenly sends us spiraling. She says to picture yourself like a pool, and in that pool are some beach balls. Each of these beach balls represents a stressor. You might be someone whose pool has relatively few balls in it. Balls might come in, but then they go out again. Such is life when we're not in a trauma response. For these people, when one more gets added, no big deal. But then there are those of us operating in functional freeze. When I was at maximum MTB, at pretty much all times my pool was packed. So when one more ball was added, it was just too much. It didn't matter whether that ball was legit stressful (like the black mold discovery) or a low-key irritant (like no hummus). Maybe you feel the same way? The way I see it, people with chronic illness—and most especially those of us with MTB—are typically functioning with a swimming pool that's 80 to 90 percent full, maybe even more, at all times.

One of the things that will often happen for me when my pool is full is that I'll get super impatient. Some internal version of me will be all arms crossed, toe tapping, thinking, *Why are you wasting my time?!* Externally, that will look like me simultaneously cooking dinner and answering an email, and when Danny bops into the kitchen all smiley and wanting to chat I'll be like, "Why are you speaking to me. Can't you see I'm *busy*?!" Typically when this happens, it's because I've been pushing myself physically, not listening to what's best for me. I know I should have cut myself some slack and ordered takeout so I could sit on the couch and rest, but I didn't honor my needs. Instead, I overrode them. The result? Too many beach balls, very little patience. At other times, I might go into more of a shut-down mode where I struggle to make even the most basic decisions.

With functional freeze, in which some part of us is essentially always in overwhelm, you can also feel numb, or like you're not sure what to do. In some cases, we look fine on the outside—like we've got it all together—but inside we're suffering.

Fun, right? But again, we don't have to stay in this space. That's the good news.

I have worked so hard on rewiring my brain and my body since the onset of my chronic illness. At this point I would say that I'm 90 percent more settled. I understand my stress response better than ever, including how to manage it when it gets disruptive to my life. In the past, when something happened it would immediately trigger my anxiety and insane fear looping. It was like the Hulk took over my brain to protect me. "Get out of way! Hulk protect

Amy!" Or Super Freak would rocket in and land on the scene. It was like I had my own dysfunctional Avengers squad!

Today, the squad's still there, but I'm in a place in my work where I can see them coming and understand that their presence is a lifesaving response that's happening in my brain. The ability to respond that way is something that's very much needed in our lives—we don't want to lose it entirely. However, at this point in my recovery, I do see that difference between what's uncomfortable and what's actually dangerous. The work is in being able to understand and live in the uncomfortable and the unknown. The reality is that something may happen to make me not feel well in the future. But then I engage my ability to trust that I, Amy, can take care of myself if something does in fact happen. (And ya know, Super Freak and the Hulk are there to back me if I need it.)

Awareness is the first step to making that transition. To taking your foot off the gas, emptying some of those beach balls from your pool, calming down your dysfunctional superheroes, and so on. We're gonna get into some of the *Hows* of doing that in part two. For now, just hold on to this idea and see how it lands with you and whether and where it resonates. That's enough.

Guess what—you made it!! We're through the trauma science and look at you. You did great! Now, be sure to stop by the booth on the way out to pick up a souvenir photo.

It's time to shift gears slightly and look at one of the biggest sources of MTB—the docs and other care providers who are supposed to be helping us. And in many cases they *are*, but, well, it's complicated.

FIVE

THE WILD, WILD WESTERN MEDICAL SYSTEM

For a long time after I got sick, I suffered with GI issues. I went to doc after doc, several of whom were reputed to be among the best in their field. Ten gastroenterologists in total and every single one of them ended up telling me some version of the same thing after running through all of their standard treatments. The responses ranged from the mundane, "I don't know. I've tried all my resources," to the shocking, "I dunno—maybe take out part of your colon?" Emphasis on the question mark. I mean, if your car was broken, how would you feel about a mechanic who said, "I dunno—maybe just take out the fuel pump?" I went from feeling safe and like the doc had a lot of tools in their toolbelt that could potentially help me, to feeling like a guinea pig, along with dismissed, unheard, and unseen.

True story: Along my journey to get relief and answers, one doc said, "I would just take it out; you will be so much happier, trust me!" She leaned in all *I got you, girl!* And she was so peppy when she said it, as if I was just clearing out an old box of knickknacks. There I was, twenty-five years old and this doc was like a medical Marie Kondo, encouraging me to toss my colon because it no longer sparked joy.

Finally, I went ahead and made an appointment to consult a surgeon, which I did out of desperation and, of course, the ongoing extreme discomfort. Thank God, he was the first person who pumped the brakes on Operation Colon. "Hmm," he said, giving me that squinty I'm-thinking-hard look. "I'm not sure that I feel comfortable doing this surgery given what you're telling me and what I'm seeing on these test results. I'd recommend that you talk to Dr. X first." The doc in question was a world-renowned expert at one of the top hospitals in the country and, fortunately for me, this surgeon could get me in with him.

So, I bundled up my faint glimmer of hope and went off to see doc number eleven, and he did a bazillion—and I mean bazillion—tests, all of which were invasive, mind you. I waited anxiously for him to come in with the results, prepped and armored that it would be another heartbreak, along with a waste of time, money, and emotional bandwidth. By that point in my health journey, that kind of bracing had become automatic. Imagine my surprise, then, when instead of dismissing me, *he fully validated and confirmed everything I felt was happening!* He literally said, "You are exactly right. Let me show you the results."

There it was. Exactly what I thought it was, and I now had the test results to prove it. Not only did he show me that exactly what I had been intuiting was true, he also confirmed that everything I was currently doing to make myself more comfortable—all the dietary tactics and holistic tools I had figured out for myself—were right on target, and he wouldn't change a thing. *IS THIS REAL LIFE? AM I IN A FEVER DREAM?* I thought.

In the end I learned that my GI problem had a neurological cause, which I'd even later learn was late-stage Lyme and the neurological damage that can come from it. Instead of surgery, this doc recommended a new drug that was in clinical trials that he was having huge success with. I said, "Sign me up!" I was like Alice in

Wonderland, happily swigging from the "drink me" cup, hoping to be transported to a magical fantasyland where people are *regular*.

The amazing news is that the drug worked for me! Until it didn't. It helped with my GI issues, but over time I could no longer ignore the increasingly large red flags that were popping up in terms of side effects. I desperately wanted to stay on this medicine because it was finally giving me relief. Still, it was irrefutable: My thyroid went wackadoodle, my liver enzymes through the roof . . . not stuff you can just brush off, or that happen out of the blue. So I went back to the doctor, by now seriously concerned. When I gave him the news about the side effects, it was like he turned into a different person. He told me, in no uncertain terms, that the dream drug had nothing to do with what I was experiencing, that the drug didn't affect other parts of the body, period.

I kind of stared at him for a minute because I couldn't quite believe what he was saying. After all, the body is a series of intricately and deeply interconnected systems. It's not really fathomable that you can take a drug and it has only one effect, in one limited area. But suddenly it was like a trapdoor opened up beneath me, and we were back to the dismissing, the belittling, and the gaslighting I'd experienced from so many other health care providers. And this time was especially painful because I thought that I'd finally found a doctor who was helping me. After all, he had believed and validated me and even had a diagnosis to back it all up. It left me reeling, causing me to doubt my instincts and question my faith in myself.

So there I was, left to deal with not only the aftermath of the medication and its side effects, but even more important, this totally unhinged, self-questioning feeling that in some ways was so much worse than the physical symptoms. That stayed imprinted on me for a very long time. It was like a ghost I couldn't escape, haunting every part of me from the inside out.

You know, as I considered what story I wanted to use to kick off this chapter, the sad thing is how difficult it was to choose. I had a list of at least fifteen stories off the top of my head that I could have told you from the front lines of this Western medical mess. And I bet you know exactly what I'm talking about because you have your own arsenal of awful experiences.

The thing is, it's not just the fault of some less-than-stellar doctors (though that's definitely a factor and one we'll talk about), it's much bigger than that. It's the system, and how it's not set up to handle chronic conditions, and it's the mindset that goes with it.

THE WESTERN MEDICAL MINDSET

The experience of seeking medical care, especially for people with chronic illness, can range from embarrassing to flat-out humiliating, from anxiety-provoking to terrifying, from frustrating to rage-sparking, and from nerve-wracking to, quite literally, trauma-inducing. To be clear, Western medicine can be both fantastic and downright miraculous at some things, like acute care, and we are lucky to have it. Got a broken bone or a huge gash in your head? They can fix that! Lifesaving interventions are their jam. Got bronchitis? They can help you. But sadly, what the system isn't as good at is providing truly patient-centered care—especially for those of us stuck in the gray, in-between places. And it's not focused on finding root causes but, instead, treating symptoms (hence the over-reliance on drugs for absolutely everything).

People with chronic illness tend to interact with the medical system more often and with more providers, and we're more likely to experience the negative extremes. *Again and again.* That's the deflating irony: that the very system that's designed to help us and in many cases truly does (I know it's saved my life on more than one occasion!) can also be the source of extremely deep and lasting wounds.

But I'm not the only one who thinks so. Michelle Hall is an expert on medical trauma, from both a clinical and a personal standpoint. In her book *Managing the Psychological Impact of Medical Trauma*, which is geared toward both physical and mental health providers, she lays out one of the central mindfucks of trauma related to your health. When I read these lines from her introduction, I felt *so seen*. Check it out: "In extreme cases of medical trauma, perpetrators are healers—they are our saviors—but when their work is done we are left to pick up the pieces of the life they have saved. Regardless of how noble the intentions, medical trauma exacts a toll that is not easily undone."

Mic drop for me. You too?

Hall opens the book with a graphic depiction of the actions her doctors took to save her life after the birth of her daughter. Yes, of course she's grateful to be alive, yet the experience also left her with a massive amount of trauma. Here's how she describes it:

> *"My own experience of medical trauma was a double-edged sword in that I felt profoundly grateful toward my health care providers . . . and at the same time was deeply troubled that my emotional health was ignored throughout my entire episode of care. The posttraumatic stress that I experienced following this trauma was the first of many dominoes to fall, and it seemed that no life domain, no relationship, no corner of my mind or cell of my body was safe from the deeply felt memory of it all. To make matters worse, as a clinical mental health counselor I mistakenly believed that it was up to me to find my own way back (or forward) to a place of vitality, hope, and healing."*

If you're like me, that really landed. If you need to take a moment to let all of that sink in, please do. It's a lot, and it hits the bullseye of what we're talking about. So it may be time to pause, do those deep breaths, have a sip of water, feel your feet on the ground, or even put the book down for the moment if you need to. Wade back in when you're ready. I'll be here, paddling around in the abyss, waiting for you.

THE LAND OF THE LOST

One of the major issues with the Western medical approach is how fractured and fragmented it is. They do what's needed in the moment, but then what? A while ago, I had knee surgery after a skiing accident. The doctor did his thing and then sent me home. I was in pain and totally out of it, which sucked, but here's the thing: That wasn't the end of the story. I had scheduled follow-ups with the doctor, I did compression and ice like they told me to, elevated it every day, and did PT twice a week until I got the all clear. In other words, *I had a plan, and that plan had an end date.*

A plan makes a patient feel empowered. Having no plan makes a patient feel lost in a never-ending dark hole. With Hall's experience (which sadly is shared by so many birthing moms), just as with patients who have chronic health issues, so often there is no plan or after-plan. You get some kind of treatment and then you're out on the curb. Good luck! (And to give credit where it's due, insurance companies play an enormous role in this.)

While healing from a torn ligament is extremely painful, you feel safe in that you hopefully trust your doctor. Plus, you know there's a standard protocol that takes place over a defined period of time. It's an approach that has worked for many before you, and you trust that it will get you to the other side. With chronic and invisible illnesses, there is no map. It's like we're wandering around the Land of the Lost. The task of trying to chart some way out is solely on our shoulders. That is an incredibly heavy weight to hold.

Again, part of it is the Western medical mindset, and part of it is that we have a "health care" system that is about disease management, rather than getting to the bottom of it all and helping you thrive. The fact is most Western practitioners look at the body like a machine, not the fantastically complex organism it is. When I spoke to Dr. Gabor Maté, he put it like this: "We live in the Western culture, which separates mind from the body, where materialism is the basic ideology. It emphasizes the physicality of things, but not the connection between things. And that's just society in general." He continued: "Imagine if we lived in a society that actually considered people's emotions. Would we be living in the world that we're living in? Would we raise kids the way we are raising them? Would we school them the way we school them? Would we treat people the way we treat them?"

I think you and I both know the answer to that: a huge NO. And that includes reducing patients to their pieces and parts. That approach has a name: reductionism. And that's exactly what materialism and reductionism do: they reduce us to objects and pieces. But the thing is, when it comes to people, our whole is so much greater than the sum of our parts.

What that means in a medical context is that you can't just change out the spark plugs and send someone on their way, yet all too often that's essentially what happens. Doctors see pieces and parts, not a whole. That means that your gastro treats your digestive system, period. Your endocrinologist addresses your hormones, period. And so on. And most of the time they don't even talk to each other. That leaves you to act as the go-between in a high-stakes version of the game Telephone.

Unless your doctors were trained in a holistic approach, it's likely that no one is stepping in to look at the interrelatedness of it all, along with the impact on your mental and emotional health (and vice versa). If we want that kind of care, we have to take it upon ourselves to find those kinds of docs, which are few and far between. Or we have to become a detective, reading articles and case studies, trying to find complementary approaches that might fill in those gaps, while simultaneously being our own care manager, disease specialist, and advocate.

Do you remember the game Plinko? There's a big board and all these pegs, and you drop a disc in the top and watch as it bounces along, zigging and zagging all the way to the bottom. You have no idea what path it'll take or where it'll come out, you're just hoping for a good result. In the Western medical system, patients with invisible illnesses are often like that disc, hitting one obstacle after another, with no idea where we'll end up or what we'll feel like when we come out the other end. We just go along and hope for the best, and that's not what providing truly caring care looks like.

One of the most painful things about all of this is how little empathy so many health care professionals seem to have. And that doesn't just hurt us emotionally, it turns out that low empathy can also negatively impact the quality of treatment we receive.

The idea of viewing the body and mind as separate shows up in a lot of places, but especially in patient care. Our physical symptoms are dealt with, but our mental and emotional experience is typically neglected. Yet, how could we not be emotionally affected by what happens with us physically? Why is it that so many patients with chronic illness feel so little empathy from doctors and the system as a whole? And why do so many of us with chronic conditions feel low empathy from our health care providers when we are the more complicated cases?

When I raised this issue with Dr. Maté, he had a powerful insight. I was describing how in so many of my interactions I've had with doctors, they felt so guarded and like they were only speaking to me from their heads. I got no sense from them that they understood, or cared, what I was actually going through. What were they guarding? "I'll tell you," he said. "Their own vulnerability. Their own traumas that they hadn't dealt with. That's why they're guarded, and that's why they're up in their heads, because to be connected to body, heart, and gut is vulnerable." Powerful, right? But if you think about it, it's so true. Connecting with someone who, themselves, is in a really vulnerable space requires some degree of vulnerability on the doctor's part. And if they're not willing or able to go there, the patient is kind of left out in the cold. Everything becomes distanced, disconnected, and clinical.

And lack of empathy from doctors doesn't just *feel* bad, it's actually linked to poor diagnostic skills. Researchers took a group of fifty primary care docs and recorded their interactions with patients, then analyzed the conversations to dissect their communication. They looked for things like whether the doctors were empathetic, whether they reassured patients, and whether they used open-ended questions—or not. The patients whose physicians showed these positive behaviors were more likely to actively engage in the conversations, and to *actively participate in their own care*. They were more likely to give their docs detailed information about what they were experiencing and express their opinions about treatment options. I've lived this firsthand.

Again, this is a system malfunction—one that doesn't just feel bad in the moment, it can contribute to real, lasting trauma. And that's the paradox at the heart of this—that people who help us are in some cases also hurting us.

THE MEDICAL TRAUMA PARADOX

I want to take a moment to clarify something that I haven't yet talked about with regard to MTB. As a term, *medical trauma* has typically meant the kind of *physical trauma* you experience related to medical issues. Like, a concussion or surgery or a heart attack. It can also relate to some of the fear or anxiety you might experience after an acute, life-threatening health episode, like a stroke.

Until pretty recently, when people talked or wrote about *medical trauma*, it was often this kind of thing. Like trauma to the body from a car accident. It could have an emotional component, but it isn't the same lingering mental-emotional trauma that I'm describing with MTB. (Though they're also not totally divorced from one another because, again, humans? We're complex and everything is interrelated.)

To be clear, MTB is that space when you're actually starting to feel better with regard to your illness, but you're struggling mentally and emotionally in this silent place. It's the hell between sick and well! The illness after the illness. But MTB and medical trauma are intertwined because if you experience MTB, you've likely also experienced some form of medical trauma.

On top of trauma (medical trauma, MTB, or otherwise), there's the insane paradox of the contradictory feelings we can have about the medical system and our providers. It's like what Michelle Hall experienced. The same things that are helping us can also hurt us—like a medication that works on your primary symptoms but causes hideous side effects. Or there's the surgeon who saves your life but is also a complete jerk to you. It's that kind of ambiguity—that trapped-between-worldness—that is such a hallmark of MTB overall.

Humans often struggle with ambiguity in any case. We, and our brains, generally prefer things to be clear and straightforward. But get this: According to researchers, people with anxiety issues tend to interpret ambiguity as *threatening*. Meaning they find a lack of clarity and certainty unnerving and even fear-inducing. Anybody else got their hand up? Both hands up for me.

Also, arguably, how could you *not* have anxiety if you are tasked to deal with all of this on your own? So, if you've got MTB, where anxiety is super common, you're even more likely to struggle with this rotten paradox. It just adds to the general combo of angst and murkiness so common to the experience.

Patients with chronic illness often wrestle with a chronic lack of clarity. The perpetual uncertainty can feel extremely unsettling (to say the least). There have been times when I've felt like I was living in a state of constant threat, and sadly the way I was treated by the system often made it worse. For people with MTB, medical "care" can be even more traumatizing. How's that for a lousy plot twist?

Remember the whole thing about nervous system dysregulation and how many mental and physical problems it can cause? Well, this kind of messed-up dynamic contributes to it. At the heart of it all (no pun intended), your nervous system *can't* regulate when you don't feel safe. And how are you going to feel safe with your provider—a space where you're extremely vulnerable—when the way they treat you leaves you feeling bad about yourself? And, when the way the system is set up leaves you always having to fight for yourself? For instance, join me as we enter the not-so-wonderful world of *medical gaslighting.*

THE WONDERFUL WORLD OF MEDICAL GASLIGHTING

Unfortunately, one of the places people most commonly experience gaslighting is in the doctor's office. But don't take my word for it. In 2024, the *American Journal of Medicine* published an article titled "Medical Gaslighting: A New Colloquialism." The article says the term is usually used to describe, "negative patient experiences of having clinical concerns inappropriately dismissed or invalidated by their attending physicians." While the authors note that the term is often overused to describe a wide range of "bad clinical experiences," they acknowledge that medical gaslighting is indeed a real thing. (That's something you and I already knew, but it's nice to see the pros tossing some validation our way.)

Harvard Medical School has an article on its website discussing medical gaslighting, which describes it as "when health care professionals seem to invalidate or ignore your concerns." They might simply flat-out tell you that you're overreacting, that it's all in your head, or one of my personal favorites, that you can't actually be feeling what you're feeling because it *doesn't make sense.* And this behavior isn't just annoying and exhausting, it can have more severe effects. According to Harvard, "It can be linked to missed diagnoses, delayed treatment, and poor health outcomes. It might damage your trust in the health care system and make you less likely to seek care." Four words: Hell. Yes. Been. There. And I'm definitely not the only one.

I came across a study of patients with Ehlers-Danlos syndrome (EDS), which can be notoriously difficult to diagnose and treat because of its far-ranging symptoms. See if the title of this paper, alone, doesn't tell you something: "Clinician-Associated Traumatization from Difficult Medical Encounters." The authors write, "Patients with hypermobile Ehlers-Danlos syndrome often experience psychological distress resulting from the perceived hostility and disinterest of their clinicians." As the researchers found, "Cumulative effects of numerous negative encounters lead patients to lose trust in their health care providers and the health care system, and to develop acute anxiety about returning to clinic to seek further care." How crushingly sad is that? And here's something else that's tragic.

Research shows that women and others in marginalized groups are more likely to experience bad doc behavior. In one survey, a staggering 72 percent of women said they experienced medical gaslighting, with 71 percent saying they have been flat-out told that they were making up or imagining their symptoms! What the actual fuck? (Remember that lovely doc o' mine who suggested that perhaps what I actually needed was a prescription for Xanax?)

Self-check! Anyone else holding your breath right now? Maybe clenching your jaw? Let's let out a collective, audible exhale.

Tennis phenom Serena Williams courageously shared her own experience of medical gaslighting after the birth of her child. Williams has a history of blood clots in her lungs, and she told a nurse that she was experiencing symptoms that felt like they were related to a pulmonary embolism. The nurse's reply? "I think all this medicine is making you talk crazy." (Yeah, it's not just doctors doing the gaslighting.) Yet as it turned out, Williams was right. Fortunately, her self-diagnosis was confirmed in time for her to receive treatment for a condition that otherwise could have been life-threatening.

Here's the thing about this behavior—whether it's gaslighting, invalidating, diminishing, condescending, or whatever the form of demeaning behavior—it doesn't just feel horrible in the moment. It evolves and compounds over time. I, for one, have a history of notoriously delayed reactions to these experiences. In the moment, it's just too intense to process everything, plus I'm trying to be a good patient. But later when I revisit the visit, I see all the nuances and assumptions. It's liked a fucked-up *Highlights* spread: "Find the Gaslighting!" And the consequences can be *deep*.

THE OH-SO-DEEP WOUND OF QUESTIONING YOURSELF

The point of all of this is not to complain about doctors or the medical system as a whole, but to understand how we ended up in MTB-Land. For me, one of the most difficult aspects of MTB is the damage to my relationship with myself. I trace that directly to my many messed-up interactions as a patient with a complicated health history functioning within a messed-up medical system.

One of the lingering effects I noticed from all of the incessant gaslighting, minimizing, and doc-splaining I experienced was that it *eroded my trust in myself.* Doctors would say all kinds of things to invalidate my experiences, but the silent messaging underneath it all came through loud and clear: I don't know how to fix you, and I don't think you know what you're talking about. Subtext: You are on your own. It's bad enough when that happens in one or two interactions with a doctor or other health care provider, but when you're someone with a chronic illness, it can happen on repeat.

As I touched on in my opening story about the gastroenterologist who turned on me, to not be believed creates a deeply painful wound. It can make you question yourself, and whether or not you even believe yourself. This is a pain point for me because I really do appreciate and respect doctors. In some cases the physicians I went to really helped me, but the truth is that most of the time I was disappointed. And get this: For far too long, I blamed this lack of positive results on myself. I figured I must be failing as a patient, or that I must be some special, extra-difficult mystery case like the kind you'd see on *House.* When they get annoyed with you or become impatient or dismissive, it's easy—especially for women—to go into self-blame mode and take it. That's a pretty messed-up dynamic, shaming yourself because your docs can't figure it out and because you don't fit into an easily defined box. And I ask you: What kind of health care is that?! And, what kind of self-care is that?

Dr. Maté had some incredible stuff to say about all of this. For starters, there's the phrase *invisible illness.* When I mentioned invisible illnesses, he asked me to stop and look at that word, "invisible." He said, "Invisible to who? It's not invisible to the patient. It's only invisible to the Western medical mind that only deals in disease categories, and only when they can do tests to identify or quantify something. They're not invisible at all to anybody who's got eyes.

And it's certain not invisible to the patient." I bet you've experienced that, too. If a symptom or experience you had wasn't validated by a lab test or some other assessment, it was invalidated.

As Dr. Maté put it: "When the doctors say, 'It's all in your head,' they mean you are imagining it. But there's no imagining. Nobody's imagining their symptoms. I mean, there are rare cases, but mostly people are experiencing those symptoms. They're real, they're not invisible at all. It's only invisible to certain techniques that are available to the Western medical mind." Breathe that in with me and let it settle for a minute. How validating is that? But that's not all!

When I told Dr. Maté how I felt like so often I hadn't been believed, he told me, "Not being believed is not a *feeling*, it's an *experience*." In other words, it wasn't my perception, it was reality. I was not believed. Period.

Yet while not being believed was intensely impactful, it wasn't the only thing that made me disconnect from myself. The other reason I lost trust in myself was just the nature of chronic illness. It's the fact that our own bodies are the source of our struggle. It can feel like some part of us is working against the other parts. For me, I grew impatient with my body and had a "Hurry up, already!" attitude toward it. That can stem from not being believed or constantly being told you're a hypochondriac, or that you're being too loud about something. But it can also be because your physical body is struggling, and the rest of you just wants to get out of this unsafe space—within your own body and within the medical system—and move on with your life.

Plus, if your experiences were anything like mine, you may have often felt rushed with your providers during office visits, which doesn't help. According to an article shared by the American Association for Physician Leadership, the average primary care doc could be responsible for *three thousand patients*! Nurses and other health care providers are dealing with similar (and sometimes additional) challenges. But then you pay the price, because it's like you take that impatience, weaponize it, and point it at yourself. But you deserve so much better, dear friend. You truly do.

Let's hit that big pause button again, dim the lights, and cue the soft music. In real time, we don't typically realize these things are happening, and we're so focused on our survival and getting better that we don't prioritize our feelings. You know this song—I've sung it in previous chapters. But let's take a second to appreciate how counterproductive it is to be so hard on yourself. You're doing the best you can. You always have been. It's not your fault that this is so tough. Don't turn away and reach for your phone, I mean it! It's really, truly, not your fault. And it's gonna get better!

And you know what? Here's the cool thing: Your body is the one that told you something was wrong in the first place. Your body was ringing the alarm for help, so it is not something to be frustrated with, it's something to be grateful for!

Still, when you have someone with a stethoscope telling you not to listen to yourself or communicating nonverbally that you are just being difficult—paired with a system that doesn't allow professionals the time to truly explore the complexity of your condition and get you better—it can be easy to go along with them. To stop fighting. We should be working together! Once again: ATMOSPHERE OF HEALING, PEOPLE! We should really try it.

It's enough to make a person pretty angry. That said, let's pull the car over for a second. I wanna have a little chat about working with that completely valid emotion.

ACKNOWLEDGING HEALTHY ANGER

Perhaps more than any other aspect of MTB, the fact of how often patients suffer from medical providers—the very people who are supposed to be helping us—not having time or energy or empathy for us *makes me angry*. Maybe it makes you angry, too. And that's a totally appropriate response! So I wanna make space for it right here, right now.

I'll tell you something, though: I wasn't always in touch with my anger. For a long time, healing was my main focus and everything else became secondary, so I suppressed those feelings. I tried to be that good patient, which entailed swallowing most of my emotions, including and especially anger. I realized as I started to process everything that I was enraged, and I had no idea. Remember the fire analogy a few chapters ago? Well, I became like an actual house on fire! It's been part of my healing—and could be part of yours, too—to be in touch with my anger and express it in healthy ways.

I mentioned earlier that in my conversation with Dr Maté, he was asking me how I felt not being believed. I literally couldn't name an emotion. We went back and forth for a minute, with Dr. Maté asking me how I felt and me not being able to identify something that was an actual emotion. Finally, I struck gold. "Angry," I said. "I felt angry." I wasn't believed, and deep down that made me *angry*. See? Now I can say it!

Anger is one of the biggest emotions that can get bottled up inside us, and it lies beneath *a lot* of trauma. Over the years and with a lot of therapy, I learned that I often mistake my anger for anxiety, because it feels less safe to express rage. So if you're feeling torqued and torched, well, good for you!

Let me be clear: I'm not encouraging you to go to your doctor's office and give them a piece of your mind or toss your raspberry bubble tea all over their white coat (though, sure, we can fantasize about it for a good long moment). There are constructive ways to address any anger you may be feeling. Plus, over time I realized that often what was underneath my anger was extreme sadness. Maybe it is for you, too. Either way, both need to be addressed.

The moral of the story is that all of that is a lot to unpack. The reality is that it takes time and patience to work through the stress and trauma caused by our interactions with the medical system and our experience of being a professional patient. But, fortunately, that's not the entire story. For every person with a chronic illness, while most of us can list a litany of negative experiences, the opposite is also true. I want to take a second (though they deserve much more) to give a shout-out to all of those absolutely incredible health care providers out there. Most of us can describe moments when we received flat-out soul-healing care and attention from absolute stars in the medical world. Pour one out for the angels! I remember these memories so vividly because they really warmed my heart and gave me hope.

It is so important, and healing, to pause periodically and feel deep, abiding gratitude for the others—those dedicated docs, nurturing nurses, and even the jovial janitors coming to clean your room who make the suck of chronic illness at least a little bit better. They're the folks who really do listen, who care, who offer a smile and some encouragement. There are also the amazing partners, friends, parents, and others in our circle who truly are there for us, offering the good love. And they are *gold.*

Whew! That was a lot to get off our chests. Let's shake it off, shall we?

In the next chapter we'll look at what else is out there, meaning health care providers who are actually attending to your health, with care.

SIX

FROM THE PASSENGER'S SEAT TO THE DRIVER'S SEAT

From an early age, we're taught to defer to people in power—to follow someone else's lead. It starts with our parents. Later, we transfer this dynamic to others—to people like teachers, police officers, and, you guessed it, doctors.

In a way it makes sense. After all, doctors went to school (a lot of it) to learn how to help patients. So we look at them as the experts. Yet while they typically have more information about a lot of things than we do, there's one thing they are not experts at, because they can't be, and that is *knowing us*. The truth is, the only expert at you, is you.

Yet we tend to give doctors all of our power. Some happily take it, but we're also the ones doing the giving. That means we, too, play a role in the power imbalance. Often, we do this because we're trying to be a good patient (and we think that's what good patients do) and we're just *so desperate* to get better. But what's truly tragic is that over time, we might actually start to believe that our opinions and feelings don't matter, and so we put them to the side. And this, my friend, is a serious problem. Not only does it lead us to lose our trust in ourselves, it actually complicates our care.

Within our current medical system, people with chronic illness don't fall into easily defined boxes. We tend to present with signs and symptoms that are confounding and at times contradictory. On top of that, one intervention may help with some things but cause other problems. Then we look to one doctor—or even a team of them—to solve all of this. But without our deep engagement, usually they can't. So all too often, they're left shooting in the dark. All the while, we're struggling, both physically and emotionally, but we're reluctant to speak up, or are discouraged from doing so. It's the perfect storm for trauma. And that's why you're out at sea, doing the best you can to tread water.

Well here's the moment you've been waiting for: it's time to start making that shift to a more empowered dynamic. Spoiler alert: only you can do that. It's time to take that driftwood you've been clinging to and build yourself a boat.

Here's the deal: Our medical system with all the insurance problems, and on and on, is what it is. We can't fix that system. Yet. Hopefully in time someone will knock some sense into the powers that be to create something better. But, we're not there yet. And the reality is, *you're* not there yet. Meaning, you're still paddling around in struggle space without those resources to give. So first, we need to get you out of the water, dried off, and cozy warm.

Right now you're in a space where, at least to some extent, you don't know what you don't know. You're accustomed to doing things this way, and being treated this way by docs, and so it's totally normalized for you. By reading this book and reflecting on these ideas, you're starting to see where there's some dysfunction at work. Recognizing that will enable you to fix the pieces that are under your control. Because when we know better, we do better.

It comes down to this: Many things about the system we're in, stink. But we can either sit around with Oscar in the trash can having a kvetch fest, or we can get up and take out the trash. We can do what we can to make the experience better for us and, you know, less stenchy. It's your choice.

In all of this, I keep thinking about someone very special to me. I share this story with you not to stay in the can and perpetuate the kvetching but to help identify something that will eventually move us forward, into a more empowered role. That's what I know Sharon would want us to do.

Sharon is a former client. I say *former* because she's no longer with us, at least on this earthly plane. Her gorgeous spirit was so strong and bright it's difficult for me to imagine that she's not still here in some way. It also feels kind of wrong to describe her as a *client*, because she became a true and sincere friend so quickly after we met. She'd been diagnosed with stage 4 ovarian cancer, and I think that's what something like that does to you. When the veil is thin, you don't mess around about love and connection, which is what it's all about in the first place.

When I met Sharon, she was on her third round of treatment at one of the best-known and most respected cancer treatment centers in the country. Afterwards, she felt totally cooked—and in a way, she was. They had successfully nuked the cancer for the third time, but she was left feeling absolutely wasted. The cancer had made her body into a war zone. Picture a battlefield after a massive conflict and that's what she felt like inside—decimated.

Sharon approached me as a health coach and patient advocate, hoping I'd be able to help her rebuild her health. She asked me if I'd accompany her to her next appointment at the cancer center, where she was scheduled to see the integrative specialist. I was eager to go, to learn, to see what the specialist at this hugely respected and revered institution had to say. What I experienced fell far short of my hopes and expectations.

There I was with my notepad, poised and ready to back Sharon up. She explained her situation beautifully and expressed that she was looking for a way to build her body back after treatment. She was seeking quality of life. She said she wanted to feel as good as possible with the time she had.

What she got in response was a whole bag a' nothin'. The renowned integrative specialist looked at her quizzically, as if she was speaking a foreign language. In the end he had very little to offer. It took everything in me to not let my jaw drop. Really? That's it?

I went into advocate mode and started asking questions: What about her basic labs—can they be run? Are there any general vitamins or other supplements she should be taking? Would an IV infusion, or a series of them, potentially help her—one of those vitamin C, B, and everything else drips? What about nutrition? What foods would help her rebuild her health?

I hoped that if I primed the pump, the specialist would be inspired to jump in with some solutions. Instead, what happened was this. (I swear, you cannot make this stuff up.) He looked at me, his head slightly cocked, and said, "Huh. We really should hire someone like you to help our patients." And he meant it. Because this world-renowned integrative specialist? *He had nothing!* And, not only did he have nothing, he didn't seem to get the importance of quality of life.

Unfortunately, that seems to be a theme throughout a lot of health care. We have disease management and SICK care, not HEALTH care. And we have a lot of specialists who focus on one part of the physical body but don't understand the imperative of teaching a patient how to live optimally *overall*. That is about thriving and longevity, and it's one of the key ways for a patient to become empowered and work their way back to health.

I went back in, and after some more prodding from me (which was slightly less gentle this time), we identified three supplements she could start with. "Aaaaaand do we . . ." I gave the doctor that long pause and encouraging look that said, *Jump in here anytime buddy!* Finally I had to fill in the blank myself: "schedule a FOLLOW UP?"

"Oh, yes," he said. "Whenever you want." I was thinking, whenever we want? What I want is for you to give Sharon something, *anything*. Long pause. "Five weeks?" He was seriously asking ME.

Sharon and I left, and after a subsequent debrief, she decided she might have more luck seeking the support of a functional medicine specialist. (We'll talk more about the difference between functional medicine and other docs in a minute.)

One obvious and sad (and IMHO, infuriating) thing here is just how woefully uneducated this doc was regarding total-body care. It was all about zapping the cancer, period. No attention to recovery, to mental and emotional well-being, or to all of the things that are within the patient's control to impact their own health. And to me, that's the big takeaway here: the total disempowerment of patients. Because the reality is, there is so much we can do to care for ourselves no matter what stage of our healing journey we are in. There is always something we can do to improve our quality of life, no matter what. But two huge things get in our way.

The first is that overall lack of understanding in our culture about the fact that the mind-brain-body are not separate. (News flash!) And we ignore these deeply interwoven connections inside us at our peril.

The second is this power differential I keep talking about, where patients view doctors almost as supreme beings who should have the ultimate say over our treatment. "Doctor knows best!" is a phrase I have heard most of my life. Not only is that dynamic not healthy, there is also such a huge chasm in knowledge and awareness for so many doctors when it comes to the world beyond surgery and drugs—the world of acute care and symptom management. If we are nowhere to be found in our healing plan, it creates a gap we then fall into.

Now, I want to take a moment to inject some more clarity here. Within all this dysfunction, we cede our power and our voice to docs, or really anyone who will take it. As a result, the true cause of our illness can go undiagnosed, we get gaslit, we feel rushed, unseen, unheard, and on, and on. And so we're forced into a self-advocacy role, but one that's exhausting. We're constantly struggling upstream like human salmon, trying to find help, and then also manage that help all by ourselves. We're advocating for ourselves, but it's not in a positive way; it's more of an emergency triage kind of approach. Cue survival stress, folks.

In the self-empowered shift I'm describing, we advocate for ourselves, but without the dysfunction. Instead, ideally, we *collaborate* with our health care providers, working like a team.

How do we do that? How do we arrive at this magical Nirvana? Well, that's what this chapter's all about! And we're going to start by owning our role in the dysfunction.

STEPPING UP TO YOUR ROLE

Here's the deal: We go to the doctor and seek care because we need help. Obviously. The mistake we make is giving all of our power to whoever we are seeing. But sometimes, let's be honest here, we also actually *want* them to have all the power. We *wish* they would just tell us what to do. I mean, wouldn't that be easier than taking an active role? Wouldn't it be easier than being responsible for our own choices?

Again, no blaming or shaming here. Far from it. I confess to having been there for a very long time myself. For a good long while it was like I was playing hot potato hoping someone would handle my illness for me.

Like most people who know there's something wrong with them but don't know what, I would have done *anything* to get well. Part of that was believing that my doctors had supernatural healing powers, which of course they did not. It's kind of like what Jungians call a *golden shadow*. Instead of owning our own innate wisdom, we see doctors as knowing more about us than we do. We're projecting our knowingness on them. But there's a payoff in that because we don't have to take responsibility for our choices. Ouch, right? I know. I didn't love it when I landed on that realization either. It was like tripping over myself and falling onto a cactus.

When I talked to Dr. Gabor Maté, he had some powerful reframing to offer. When I asked him what he'd say to people who experienced this—who gave over their power to doctors and therefore lost trust in themselves—he said this: "First of all, they need to understand that the loss of trust in themselves wasn't a mistake on their part. It was actually a survival mechanism."

This gets back to what I said earlier: that from an early age, we're taught to defer to people in power. Typically, this starts with our first caregivers. When we're peanuts, we can't care for ourselves, so in a very real sense, we *need* those people to survive. That means that when they act like jerks—doing things like dismissing us or invalidating our feelings—we figure out ways to suppress ourselves or otherwise behave in ways that keep us connected to them. Then, as we get older, we can transfer this dysfunctional pattern to doctors. We need their help to get better, so in our deepest thinking (often at the level of the unconscious), some part of us desperately seeks to maintain that connection. These interactions with doctors can ping that trauma pattern in your brain-body from earlier in life, essentially reactivating it in real time.

That's what Dr. Maté meant when he used the phrase *survival mechanism*. As he characterized it to me, it's "choosing attachment over authenticity." Meaning, you're doing what you need to do to stay connected to that other person instead of being authentic to yourself—expressing your true thoughts, advocating for yourself, and so on—and risking that they'll disengage from you. *That*, my friend, is what it means to put on a mask. (And if you want to learn about the idea of attachment versus authenticity in more detail, I highly recommend Dr. Maté's book *The Myth of Normal*.)

But let's circle back to the first part of what he said because it is so important. That putting on the mask and choosing attachment over authenticity *wasn't a mistake on your part*. You were doing what you needed to do in the moment because of the limited resources available to you. You see, when you're in all-out survival stress mode, you're going to invoke survival mechanisms. You don't have a lot of access to higher-level thinking and resources.

Over time I realized that having faith in doctors was just that—faith. We want someone to save us, to figure it all out for us because we think it will be easier that way, and it's too painful to deal with alone. Add to the equation the fact that you're probably drained of energy and cognitive capacity and the idea of throwing it all to someone else to take care of is extra appealing. After all, you've got nothin' in the tank. I know, I get it. We're at a loss for how else to handle our health. We don't know another way, and we don't have the energy to try to find one. You can feel so helpless that you forget that you, my friend, are a critical part of the equation. Doctors are a lot of wonderful things, but a magical and all-healing wizard (or witch) is not one of them.

But now, things are different. As your symptoms become more manageable and the survival stress begins to calm down, you're getting more capacity and becoming more resourced. That means you have more tools available to you to handle things differently. To choose authenticity.

And here's the thing, gang: You got some serious stuff *right* in the past. Guess who knew that something was wrong in the first place? You! You are that smartie. You did that. So you aren't exactly chopped liver sitting over there. You are pretty wise and intelligent and knew enough to go get help in the first place. That seems like a valuable partner to me. Just sayin'.

Lemme drop some scary and empowering math on you: We are 50 percent of our healing team, and we are 100 percent responsible for how we treat ourselves.

Again, this realization is meant to be empowering. It's not about the past—forget about that for the moment. Take the lessons and move on. We're right here, right now, standing here with all these pieces of wood and screws and manuals that make no sense, figuring out how to assemble your boat.

Here's the shift: When you look at finding a doctor as less about finding someone who will give you straight-up answers and more about finding a partner in your health, that's when the balance of power tips in your favor. Chronic illness is not easy: there is no magic bullet. If there were, the disease rate would not be so high.

Earlier in the book, I mentioned a client of mine who has hemiplegic migraines. She has been through so much and has seen so many doctors that it's hard to keep track of them. One doc she was seeing treated her with Botox, which is a fairly common short-term remedy for migraines. Side note: He's the head specialist at one of the best-known headache centers in the country. In other words, he's the dude.

The doctor who prescribed the injections believed my client's pain had nothing to do with anything that was happening elsewhere in her body. She told me this particular doctor made her feel anxious and scared. He was sarcastic with her and laughed at her questions. When she complained to him about weight gain, he told her that it was due to "a food intake problem." In other words, she eats too much. (I wish this kind of shitty talk was rare, but on top of experiencing it myself, I also hear about it a lot from others.) Later, it was determined that my client's weight gain was actually a side effect of a medication she was taking.

When doctor-patient interactions get like this, it's like any toxic relationship. It's hard to cut off, but it feels necessary for your health. But the point is, *you have to make that move.* You have to get in the driver's seat, fire their ass, and find someone else. (I know in some cases that's easier said than done, and we'll talk about some of those challenges in a minute.)

I just want to say this again because it's so important: I really do not want to give the impression that I think all doctors are insensitive and unaware. That's definitely not true. And multiple times, doctors have saved my life. And many more times they have been very kind to me, regardless of whether their care fell short or not. In other words, they've given me the best they've got. And let's face it—their job isn't easy. Not by a long shot. Yet neither is dealing with a chronic illness. Again, it comes back to this black-and-white way of looking at things. And we, my friends, are in the gray zone. And that's why it's important to, if you can, try to find the health care providers who will truly care for your overall health and healing.

Patients who suffer with chronic illness need someone on their team who is looking at the whole situation holistically. If we don't have what we need within the system, we have to go out and find it for ourselves, otherwise we're free-falling. It's like we have to create our own parachute. Because who the hell wants to be hurtling through space without one? Literally no one.

Let's be real—doctors are extremely important. They play a critical role in our health care. We need them for diagnosis and for their expertise in helping to give us information that will help us make the best choices for us. Ideally, that's how we're working with our health care providers: as a team.

All of that said, what does one of those 50/50 doctor-patient relationships look like? I found out when I met my current doc. (Cue the gauzy, soft-focus camera: It's flashback time!)

A NEW KIND OF DOC-PATIENT RELATIONSHIP

Sometimes you find a doc who not only gets *you* but gets *it*. For me, Dr. Leo Galland is that person. In my experience, he's the perfect example of a physician who provides not only sound medical advice but also something else that makes such a huge difference: empathy! He has been in the trenches with me all the way from deep sickness through to my escape from The Shadowlands. He told me and affirmed for me, "Being sick alters your sense of who you are and regaining your health helps you become a different self."

It's been through my relationship with Dr. Galland that I've learned the power of agency. Of being actively involved in my own care and taking responsibility for my own choices. As I've come to believe, the more a person is engaged in their care, the more therapeutic the process is. If you're simply the passive object of a doctor's treatment and you manage to get better, that's good. There's real value in the outcome. But when you're actively involved in your treatment, it's not just about treatment, it's about empowerment.

As patients, we sacrifice so much when we get sick, and in many cases we lose our identity as we knew it. This type of care empowers you to step back into your body, and into your life, to believe that you have the answers. That you are capable of trusting yourself and getting yourself better. That you have the ability to step up and save yourself. To build that boat!

As I discovered, being so deeply involved actually helped me heal other wounds—those that had been created by my previous interactions with other health providers. I began to learn to trust myself again. To take off my mask and be myself. To admit that I was hurting in other ways from the whole experience, not just physically. To stop second guessing or trying to be the good patient. Because I realized that the best patient is (say it loud and proud with me) an empowered one.

That's on the patient side, but what makes for a good doctor? A good doctor is one who practices empathy, flexibility, thinks outside the box, and has immense wisdom. But that's not all. A good doctor—the best kind—sees their role as affirming their patients. They encourage, and even require, you to be an active participant in your care.

I was lucky to find that in Dr. Galland, but I gotta say, it was uncomfortable at first. It was a completely different dynamic from what I'd experienced to that point. I had to take baby steps, and for a while I kept looking to him for reassurance that it really was okay for me to speak up, to toss out ideas, and to make decisions for myself. It felt so foreign to have him ask me what I thought about something, or the idea that he even wanted my feedback to help inform his decisions. It was like I was a kid in rainboots, tentatively dipping my toes into a puddle and looking up to make sure it was okay for me to splash.

I sought him out hoping against hope that he could diagnose me correctly. I went to him for his knowledge, his reputation, and because I needed a doctor to help me find answers and a path forward, so that I could help myself. I had been a damn good water treader, but I wanted out of that pool. After he landed on the correct diagnosis, Dr. Galland shared that while he was there to support me through my treatment—and shift gears if we needed to—the work, the schedule, and the speed at which we engaged was ultimately up to me. It was both refreshing and wince-inducing all at once. Really? I get to/have to be a big girl, stepping into my power and making informed decisions for my own body? *Gulp.* Inside, my Good Patient squeaked, "But, *you're* the doctor." I had so much to unlearn. And so much to learn.

For background, Dr. Galland is an integrative medicine doctor. Functional/integrative docs are different in that they take a much more holistic approach than typical Western docs. They're like Western docs *plus.* They treat you if you need acute help. But if you've got a persistent pain in your lower back, they're not just going to look at your lower back. They're going way deeper, to anything that could potentially influence what you're experiencing. Their goal is to get to the root, and to treat the whole person. So while they might prescribe medication for something, they might also suggest dietary changes, exercise, mental health interventions, and so on. Actual fun fact: It was Dr. Galland who recommended I add EMDR—a therapy focused on trauma and distressing life experiences—to my protocol. Imagine that!

As I was working on the book, I had this conversation with Dr. Galland that underscored what I'm talking about. It was all about helping you, dear reader! He said that in his entire career, he's never separated the mental from the physical. Then he said that amazing thing about how regaining your health helps you become a different self. As he explained, the way he sees it, our mental-emotional health is just as important to overall health as what your blood pressure is or how your labs look.

Dr. Galland shared with me a conversation he had with a friend of his who is a cognitive behavioral therapist. The therapist said to him, "What you're doing with your patients is psychotherapy." Dr. Galland said he didn't see it that way because he wasn't psychologizing with people. But the therapist persisted, explaining that any time you help people "solve their way to health" (I love that piece), it's psychotherapy. And I'm sharing that because I want you to have that concept in your own mind—the idea of *solving your way to health.*

My doctor told me that, when it comes down to it, he wants to help create empowered patients. He said, "I know I did a good job when someone says to themselves, 'What would Dr. Galland tell me to do?'" It's not because he knows best, but because they're acting as their *own* version of him. They're thinking through what's best for them and trusting themselves to be right about it. As Dr. Galland told me, "The origin of the word 'doctor' is *teacher* or *leader*, and that's the role I like to be able to fill."

It was actually Dr. Galland who said to me, "Amy, from my perspective, the hardest thing about what you're going through is that you don't trust yourself." He then gave me examples of that, and I could see it clear as day. That rang so true in me it was like a giant gong going BONG and reverberating all throughout my brain-body.

As I write about this, another analogy comes to mind. It's like you and your doctor are solving a puzzle together. Maybe you lock down the border, and your doc comes in with some of those hard-to-find, weird-shaped pieces. The point is, you each have some of the pieces. You each bring something important to the table. But it's always clear that it's *your* puzzle, and you steer the puzzle-solving ship. Dr. Mark Hyman put it this way during a podcast interview: "Most of your health is not happening in the doctor's office. Eighty to ninety percent of it happens with things that you can have control over. It happens in your kitchen. It happens where you play and eat and pray and work. That's where health happens. It's the environment that you live in and it's your choices every day. Those things you don't really need health care for." But it's on you to take that initiative. No doctor can get you to jump in and do your part—only you can do that.

Early in our relationship, even when I tried to slip into that passenger seat, Dr. Galland was like, "Nuh-uh," and waved me over to take the wheel. To be clear, he never let me drive alone. He's always been right there. We just know who is running the show. And that has been nothing short of life changing. Life *saving*, in fact.

The good news is that there are some really great doctors out there. Remember my client with hemiplegic migraines? Well, there was good news for her, too. Together, we ditched the head specialist and found a functional medicine neurologist—a doctor who incorporates the principles of functional neurology. He focuses on supporting the entire nervous system by providing specific neurological exercises and stimulation. My client was so excited to find him. And it's been satisfying for me to watch her metabolize the understanding that she doesn't have to just take terrible from doctors. She doesn't have to twist herself and tolerate behavior she would not accept from anyone else in her life just because the person she was seeing is wearing a white coat and has a string of letters after his name and because someone once referred to him as "the best." Clearly, not the best.

So, how do *you* get out of the disempowerment trap and move into a glorious new empowered you who's jingling the keys and is ready to drive? Well, we're gonna talk about it in part two. And guess what? We're there!

Before we move on, I wanna take a minute to acknowledge all that you have done to get here. We've already been through a lot together, you and me. That was one long, dark cave. Now here we are with our clothes covered in bat guano and a bad case of head-lamp hair, but we did it! YOU did it. And that was no small thing. So, for real, take a deep breath (maybe a few) and pat yourself on your back. You made it through the cave. Let there be light!

Now that you have the science and the background, frame-work, and context of MTB, it's finally time to move on to the SOLUTIONS! Grab your captain's hat and let's go.

PART TWO

TOOLS FOR HEALING

SEVEN

RIDING THE WAVE

Here we are! We've emerged from the cave of part one into the bright, crisp dawn of part two. Smell that fresh morning air and feel the sun on your face. This is where we start healing! I'll actually let you in on a little secret. You ready? Lean in close. . . . *Your healing has already begun.*

That's right. All the heaviness and hard truths you grappled with in part one were actually the first steps on the road to recovery, and a healthier, happier future. Or at least one that's more regulated, where you're not at the mercy of MTB.

In this part of the book, you're going to learn about some of the tools that will take you even further. Because here's the thing: Remember how one of the reasons we develop MTB is the lack of a recovery plan—one that addresses trauma and the illness after the illness? Well guess what? *Here is the plan that you never got*!

Drift no more, my friend. No longer do you have to fear the waves because now you're going to learn how to ride them. Not just endure them, but proactively navigate through them, charting your own course, sailing your own ship.

Now, I'm gonna be real with you: Healing trauma and literally reprogramming your brain isn't easy. And it's definitely not fast. This is going to take some real time and some real investment in yourself. But the good news is that you're not just aiming to recover, or just get back to normal. We're going bigger than that, to a place that in some ways is better than where you were before.

And here's some more good news: while true, deep healing can take a long time, you can actually start feeling better—and I mean much better—pretty quickly. In fact, when you start implementing these tools, you could notice some changes right away. Just the awareness that you're no longer lost or spinning in circles, that you finally have a map, can give you an initial boost all by itself.

If you're like me, at least once in your chronic illness journey—and maybe multiple times—you've experienced an *epiphany paradox*. That's my lingo for a double-sided revelation, kinda like a dark cloud with a silver lining. Danny dropping the trauma bomb on me at dinner is an example. On one hand, I was knocked low by the recognition that I'd endured serious trauma and it was now stuck in my system. But on the other hand, being able to name what I was experiencing was a revelation, because it meant now I could do something about it. It's like when I got my diagnosis of late-stage neurological Lyme with multiple co-infections. No one's chest bumping or high-fiving when they discover that they have something like that. But finally knowing what's going on? That's priceless! Because now you know what you're working with and can see that there is, indeed, a light at the end of the tunnel. So yeah, you have MTB. That's the yucky realization. And, here's your path out!

The other thing that I think is powerful about healing from just about anything is that you grow in the process. That's certainly true of trauma. There's even a name for it: *post-traumatic growth*. It means that you use trauma as a springboard into a new way of being. That means that in some ways, you can come out the other side even stronger, with greater wisdom and a new perspective. But post-traumatic growth doesn't just happen, you have to really, fully *do* the healing process. To be clear, I'm not trying to sugarcoat it. The reality is that trauma *sucks*. Yet it can also be a catalyst for good things, and that's where we're headed.

As you set out on your MTB healing journey, I encourage you to observe some basic rules of the road:

1. **Easy does it.** Instead of diving in headfirst with, say, six days in a row of intensive sauna, or signing up for a two-week silent meditation retreat when you've never meditated before, *start slow*. Dip your toe in the proverbial pool first so you can see how your brain-body responds and you don't risk overdoing it.
2. **Don't take my word for it.** What I'm giving you here is my best advice based on my own sphere of awareness, but there is so much more out there. There's more detailed information available about all of the modalities that I will describe, and there are also more tools and approaches than I'll cover in this book. Remember that part of your healing is becoming more empowered, and that starts NOW. I encourage you to do your own research: read articles and studies from reliable sources, talk to trusted friends and reputable providers, and so on. And a word to the wise: AI ain't all that yet. It can be easy to just go with whatever amalgamation of information our robot overlords spit out at you in response to your search, but at least for now, many of these results are either inaccurate or don't show the full picture. So, when it comes to trying something new, do your due diligence first by

investigating it thoroughly. Not just what are the potential benefits, but what are the potential drawbacks? Who is it recommended for and not recommended for? That counts double for more intensive modalities, such as cold plunging or psychedelic-assisted therapy.

3. **Be accountable.** This is kind of a follow-on of number two. Please, please, please don't do something because I or anyone else encourages you to do it if it doesn't feel right for you. You know your body best, and if something doesn't pass the smell test, don't do it! Seriously, my friend, I can't stress this enough: You have been through years of other people supposedly knowing what's best for your body when sometimes it wasn't. You've probably swallowed it down and not spoken up for or advocated for yourself. That's not a judgment. We all do it. I've done it *so many times.* But we're not doing it anymore, m'kay? This can be a really hard habit to break, but it's time to find your voice. You will probably need to build that practice over time, but start practicing now, by being your own best judge of what to try and when. Deal?

Okay, now that we've got that established, let's rock! Time for the first stop on our healing voyage.

LET'S GET REGULATED

As you'll no doubt recall, we spent a bunch of time in part one unpacking some of the basic science of trauma. What we uncovered was that at the root of many of the trauma symptoms we can experience—the anxiety, fear looping, disassociation, plus all the physical stuff—lies a central problem: a dysregulated nervous system. When your nervous system is chronically dysregulated, it's like having a house that's built on a cracked foundation. It's going to cause problems throughout the structure. You can do all kinds of home renovations to fix the cracking plaster, the plumbing issues, and so on, but unless you repair that foundation, you're going to be spending half your time hunting for a good contractor.

When your nervous system is chronically dysregulated, one of the things that can happen is that you swing into fight-flight-freeze at the drop of the hat. When you begin to get more regulated, you start to have fewer swings, and when you do get off-kilter, it becomes easier to return to center.

It will come as no big surprise then that to heal MTB, you're looking to re-regulate your nervous system. As Irene Lyon framed it when we spoke, it's about moving your system out of survival stress. She described how when babies are well cared for—they're picked up when they cry, they're safe and protected, they have food, fun, engagement, movement—as they get older their nervous system begins to self-regulate. They're not relying on their caregiver to help stabilize their system. "And that's exactly what we're doing as adults when we're healing from, say, a trauma," she said. "I like to look at it as we're going back to the roots of what we needed when we were young. To be able to rewrite and rewire [our nervous system]."

So, here's the million-dollar question: *How* do you re-regulate your nervous system? Well, there are multiple approaches and entire books by clinical experts focused entirely on that question. And, there's not just one thing to do, or one framework.

That said, there are some basics that I've really liked working with because they're both simple and gentle. And, you kinda' can't go wrong with that approach because it's the safest.

Again, nervous system regulation is a project. Going back to the house idea, it's a major remodel, so it will take some time. I keep emphasizing that because I think our culture likes to go for quick and easy fixes, and it's kind of wired into us to look for that. Yet when it comes to this work, it's slow and steady that wins the race. And in fact, going too hard too fast—like, say, heading to the jungles of Peru for a six-day ayahuasca journey when you've done no prep work—could have an effect akin to dropping a bomb on your nervous system.

In fact, "too much, too fast" of *anything* is actually a setup for more trauma. And if you're anything like me, too much, too fast, has kind of been the name of the game until this point.

So, rule of thumb: Easy does it.

This idea actually brings us to one of the foundational healing concepts for MTB, which is *titration*.

EASY DOES IT: TITRATION

The godfather of Somatic Experiencing® (SE™) is a man named Peter Levine. (You might remember me mentioning him and his book *Waking the Tiger* in part one.) SE, if you're not familiar, is a trauma-healing modality focused on the idea of altering our stress response system. To do that, we go deep—down into the boiler room of our brain-body. There, we work with very basic tools to assist us in reprogramming our nervous system on a fundamental level. One such tool is called *titration*.

In a minute, we're going to talk about defusing your stress response. You can think of titration as an essential tool for that work, and as a cornerstone in your re-regulation practice. Maybe you recognize that word from another context, like your high school chemistry class. That's where Dr. Levine got the concept—from chemistry.

Picture it: You're in class, wearing those swaggy safety goggles, bent over a stand of test tubes with a pipette in your hand, titrating away. When you titrate a mixture, you're converting it from one form to another, and to do that, you take whatever's in the pipette and add *a drop at a time*. What you don't do is take a whole beaker full of one thing and dump it into the other, because it might explode in your face. Don't worry about the periodic table or anything else from chemistry class (I sure don't!). That's all you have to know: the concept of *one drop at a time*.

In a second, we're going to start looking at how you can begin to rejigger your stress response so it doesn't launch you into a full-blown triggered trauma rodeo. The idea with titration is that as you approach this kind of trauma work, you want to go drop by drop. Bit by bit. Exposing yourself a little at a time. Taking small bites. Whatever language resonates with you. This is not "Go big or go home!" time. This is "Go very, very slow, even if it feels unnatural at first" time.

So if something starts to feel like it's too much, if things start to feel like they're ramping up in your nervous system, dial it back. Engage your tools (which we'll start to get into in a moment) until that stress needle starts to go back down into the green zone. In fact, if you only remember three words out of this entire chapter, remember these: EASY DOES IT.

You know, when I was a kid, I was the slowest balance beam walker of all time. I could have won a medal, I'm not kidding. I would go to birthday parties where the beam had a foam pit the size of a swimming pool surrounding it, and I was so cautious I'd cause a backup with a line all the way around the foam pit. Now, Big Amy wishes she could go back and assure Little Amy that the worst that could happen was that she would fall into a foam pit. Still, I gotta respect that little nugget's commitment to being cautious when trying new activities. And in this case, let's follow Little Amy's lead.

The cool thing is that this phase of the process is a really great opportunity to get to know yourself in a different and deeper way. You'll discover what works for you and what doesn't, your strengths and sensitivities, and so on.

Okay, ready to ease in? Get out your big toe—it's time to dip!

THE FOUR *RS* AND REPROGRAMMING YOUR STRESS RESPONSE

Did you see that movie *The Hurt Locker*, about army dudes who defuse bombs? Well grab your fatigues and your blast gear because you're about to become the next Jeremy Renner as we learn how to defuse your stress response. To underscore from part one, your stress response isn't a bad thing. It can save your life. We're not trying to totally unplug it. We just want to balance it out so it's less likely to overreact. In other words, don't clip the red or the black one!

I know for me, one of the biggest triggers of my stress response—in the wild, fear-looping MTB way—is anything that prompts me to frantically question, "*Am I getting sick again?*" Or, "*Could this make me as sick as I was before?*"

Maybe the same is true of you, or perhaps it's something else. Either way, before you rev the motor from 0 to 100, before that familiar feeling of dread arises, before the wave hits, you need to have a plan.

Remember the old saying, "Stop, drop, and roll!" It was the fire-response mantra they always told us at school. With MTB, the fire threat is high, so similarly, you want to have an advance plan of what to do when you start to get triggered. You want to have a go-to process for how to defuse that response before it kicks into high gear.

To help you devise your plan and put it into action, I've come up with the Four *R*s. And they go a little something like this . . .

Step One: Ready

First things first: a good scout is always prepared. Before I feel that full-blown stress response in my body, i.e., when the water starts to warm up, I engage my plan to turn down the heat. This means that first you have to know how to tune into your body enough to recognize the early-onset indications that your stress response is gearing up.

For me, my heart starts to speed up and I feel prickles spreading through my body. Or, I recognize that I went from fine to hopping on the worry train to nowhere good in five seconds flat, and my brain is starting to do its thing of rapidly cycling through worst-case scenarios.

That is where stop, drop, and roll comes in. At the first sign of struggle, I turn to SUDS. SUDS stands for the Subjective Units of Distress Scale, and it's a tool from cognitive behavioral therapy (CBT). It involves rating the level of distress you're experiencing on a scale of 1 to 10, where 0 is no distress and 10 is what-the-fuck-the-wheels-are-totally-off! (Apparently the clinical term for that is *extreme distress.*)

How high I am on the scale determines the action I take. Yet at the same time, just rating yourself is, in a way, its own tool. That's because when you take a minute to step back and assess how you're feeling and what's going on in your brain-body, it starts to shift your brain away from the emotional and reactive space and more toward the logic zone, where you can engage some perspective, and some amount of control over your feelings and reactions. You're already starting to shift out of reactivity.

When I was working on this book I interviewed CBT therapist Dr. Lindsay Tulchin, and as she explained, that's one of the primary goals of CBT: to create a space around the stress spike. You're not necessarily trying to make your distress or your anxiety go away—though wouldn't that be amazing—you're trying to increase your *distress tolerance*. You may recall that Irene Lyon used similar language in chapter 3 when she talked about the need to increase our *window of tolerance* in our nervous system. That's our ability to deal with stressors.

As Dr. Tulchin explained, when our distress level is high, it's because something unnecessarily sent us into fight-flight mode. And in this space we literally have tunnel vision. It's hard to see or feel anything beyond anxiety or fear or whatever else is going on in your particular stress cocktail. So the tools we engage in this space are aimed at dialing all of that down and broadening our vision so we can get a more accurate sense of what's happening, and see that we don't actually need to fight or flee.

What are some other simple things that make you feel better? If it helps, make a list. Is it a cup of that strangely good herbal tea from the shop down the street? Is it a warm bath? Is it scrolling through pics of your kids or cats, listening to a favorite song that always hits you right in the sweet spot, or three deep belly breaths? Start to pay attention because, again, chances are you have tools you're already using. Beyond that, try stuff. Maybe even ask your friends what they do when they're starting to feel overwhelmed.

Step Two: Routine

Once I've SUDS'd myself, I turn to the routine that helps *redirect* me. Here's the deal: You gotta leave the scene of the crime, and in this case, that scene is your mind. I'm not saying you check out, but instead that you refocus and reorient. And to do that you'll link some tools I'll share with you now into a routine you can turn to. These tools will be particular to you and will take some learning, though I bet you already have a few go-tos without necessarily realizing it.

One of the tools is *orienting*. It's super simple. When you feel the warning signs, orient to your surroundings. You might orient to your body—feeling your feet on the floor or your butt in the chair. Noticing something that you hear, smell, or taste (like that last sip of latte you just took). Feeling the breath enter and leave your body, and noticing your lungs expand and contract.

Once you're grounded inside yourself, you can orient to your surroundings. Check out the drawing your kid made that you tacked up on the wall. Look out the window at the curious cloud formations. It could be as simple as naming one thing you see, one thing you smell, one thing you hear, and one thing you taste. That alone could be your break. You see, orienting is about bringing your attention to the present moment, and that's one of the most powerful ways to get out of the time-warping and *what-if*–ing that can happen when we're starting to get off-kilter.

Yet the most important component of this step is the pause. You want to slow time down enough that you can create that gap between stimulus and response. And that might include creating actual distance by walking away for a minute, because where you are in that moment is just too stimulus-y.

Remember my friend Simon? He was the one dealing with long COVID. His stress response sometimes makes him want to fight with people. Simon told me when he feels anger coming on, he hops in the shower and repeats the mantra, "I am in no place to evaluate reality. I am in no place to evaluate reality. I cannot trust my mind right now. I am not in the fight any longer, I am in flight, and I am looking for a way to get out."

Self-touch and self-talk can also be remarkably effective. Have you ever seen a little kid at the playground run to a caregiver for comfort? They're crying like it's the end of the world, in a total meltdown. But insert a hug, a little back rub, and some soothing words, and thirty seconds later they're back on the slides, laughing like nothing ever happened. When we're young, we're totally reliant on others to help us re-regulate our nervous systems. When we're older, though, some of these same simple interventions can help us re-regulate ourselves. For instance, you can give yourself a hug and rub your own arms or shoulders for a few moments. For me, I automatically start massaging my scalp, which is something that totally soothed me when I was a peanut. What helps you? If you've never tried self-soothing, experiment. See if some gentle self-touch or self-talk helps to dial down your distress, even just a little bit.

Take some time to experiment with what helps you pause and redirect. Maybe it's going for a quick walk. Maybe it's splashing cold water on your face. Once you've tested out a few, make a list on a piece of paper or in the notes app in your phone that you can quickly reference.

Now that you have some tools, we'll link a few together to create the routine for redirection. For example, you might turn to a mantra, like Simon does. Say something like, "I'm okay. Everything is okay." Once the needle starts to nudge you down your SUDS scale, you add something else. You go for a quick walk, sing a song. As you're moving further down the scale, you add in one more tool, like rubbing your hands up and down your arms as if you're giving yourself a hug. This now becomes your own stress-soothing routine that you can turn to when you're feeling triggered.

One tool with a built-in routine is the rubber band technique. There are variations, and you can riff on this, but here's my version of the basic formula:

1. Wear a rubber band on your wrist. (Functional, and fashionable?)

2. When you start to notice the stress response, snap it! That's your cue to shift gears into the rest of the routine.
3. After you've snapped the rubber band, say, "Stop—snap out of it!" to yourself. (With kindness, you're not reading yourself the riot act.)
4. Next, picture a big red STOP sign halting you in your tracks.
5. Take a few big deep breaths.
6. Have a sip of water if you have some nearby.
7. And close by making a vocalization such as "Aaah" or "Hmm." The vocalization creates a vibration that signals to the vagus nerve (part of your nervous system that plays a major role in helping you down-regulate) that you're safe.

Step Three: Reality Check

The first two steps help to take the edge off, dialing down that highest level of overexcitement. But you might still be agitated, or in an irrational space. If so, it's time to do a reality check to determine whether you're in a more manageable, rational space. It's time to pan back and take a fresh look—to redefine the moment and see things as they really are. It's about getting some perspective. Another way to think about it is that you're challenging your narrative about the situation to see if it is accurate.

Simon's story reminded me of something I sometimes do with Danny that might also be useful for you. When I know I'm in that irrational place—the one where Super Freak be full-on Super Freakin'—I'll sometimes tap Danny in and ask him, "Am I overreacting here? Because part of me wants to go down to the pharmacy right now, find that smug SOB who just told me they're not handling my compounding *starting yesterday*, and give him a piece of my mind!" Danny will shake his head in his levelheaded calm, Danny way, and say his version of, "Yeah, that's not your best idea.

Maybe don't do that." (Cut to Danny gently nudging a bowl of ice water toward me.)

When I don't have a Danny or a friend handy to help me assess, I turn to my phone. I keep an SOS list on my notes app and it includes a list of questions I can ask myself to do a reality self-check. You can use these same questions or come up with your own.

- Am I feeling supercharged, like this situation is an emergency?
- Am I feeling impulsive?
- Is my mind spinning?
- Will this be a big deal in two hours, two days, or two months?

The thing is that this action is only partially about your actual answers. It's more about *the act of asking*, which on its own requires that you move into a calmer part of your brain. And there's one more question:

- Is this an actual emergency—as in, is this a *life-threatening* situation?

As you've probably guessed, 9.999 times out of 10, for me the answer is a solid NO, and that acknowledgment dials down my excitement even further.

Going through this exercise is about asking yourself, "What's really going on here?" It's about fact-checking yourself. As Dr. Tulchin explained, it starts with identifying what you're thinking, and then talking back to your thoughts. You might say something to yourself like, "This isn't a fact, it's a feeling." Again, that starts to shift your brain from a more emotional space to a more thinking space. Remember that when we go stress-crazy, what's happening is that we're about to unleash a full-blown dose of *survival stress* into our brain-bodies. Part of us feels like there is some kind of threat present, and we need to hold our horses, stop, and evaluate whether that's true.

Another method I like when I want to question my reality is the "maybes" from CBT. I have a history of going to the worst-case scenario in my worries. You too? Maybe the person next to you in the produce section just sneezed all over the golden kiwis and you are about to launch into full-blown fear loop. *Oh my God, they look pale. What do they have? Is it plague? I bet it's plague. I just read that prairie dogs in Colorado are carriers!*

Whoooaa, girl. It's time for a reality check. The "maybes," as I now affectionately call them, are about flipping and reversing my fears. Here's an example, "Maybe that person has a hideous, highly contagious disease." Flipped and reversed it could be, "Maybe they have allergies," or "Maybe I should become a comedian. I mean seriously: prairie dogs? That's gold!" So if you're checking your reality and it's not totally adding up, ask yourself, "What else might be true?" And have fun with it if you can! Remember: It's *not* about dismissing yourself or making yourself feel silly. It *is* about assessing your reaction and maybe employing a little humor where you can. Once you've identified that the world is not actually coming to an end, you can move to step four.

Step Four: Reframe

After you recognize that your version of reality and your initial reaction were a bit skewed, you can open your eyes to what actually is and gauge an appropriate response. Of course you don't want to catch what Sneezy has (if they even have anything). However, are you about to die of some Renaissance-era illness? Probably not. So, go ahead and wash your hands thoroughly when you get home, take some extra vitamin C—that kind of thing. Do NOT start doom scrolling through WebMD looking up plague symptoms.

The key is, once again, time. It comes back to slowing things down so you can make that mental shift. Reframing involves trusting your ability to handle things. You were already next to the sneezer, that happened. What's done is done. When you go fear looping, you're worried that you need to prevent the worst thing from happening. However, whatever it is they have is already airborne. If you were exposed to a few viral particles, you can handle it. After all, in the process of managing chronic illness you've developed some mad skills. You're not helpless, you're capable. You got this!

Or maybe the best response is no response, at least for now. In my own mind, I have a one-hour rule. When I'm in that worked-up space, if I'm inclined to do something stress-motivated, I force myself to wait at least one hour. I mean if you think about it, pretty much anything can wait an hour. As Dr. Tulchin explained, even if we don't engage any other tools, over time most of our distress will fade on its own. And we're not talking days or hours, we're talking minutes. For me, a good hour tends to do the trick. For you, it might be less.

Set a timer if you need to, and while you're waiting, lean on your tools. Do a routine. When that timer dings, chances are things will have settled, at least a bit, and you won't feel the need to jump into action anymore.

Still, when the chemicals start releasing and that adrenaline gets into your system, doing *something* might be helpful. That's where a walk or some other exercise, or playing an instrument, or something else physical might feel good. Maybe even going off by yourself and having a good yell, or cry. (Not that you need to cry alone, but some people are more comfortable letting loose in private.) The point is, you might wanna *move that energy* so it's not rattling around in your system like a pinball.

Another reframing tool I like is called *acting as if.* I'll ask myself what I'd do if I wasn't overreacting. "If I *wasn't* being Super Freak right now, how would I respond?" Then I fake it till I make it, acting as if I have a totally regulated nervous system. Nothing to see here, folks! I'm orienting, I'm titrating . . . All good! In other words, you don't actually have to get your internal space all flowy and calm before you act. Sometimes, emotion follows action, and that soothing calm can come later. I often find that's the case when I choose to wait an hour. I feel wired and fried at first, but after making the choice to wait, the good vibes arrive on the next bus.

These are some basics to get you started. And, I've found that it's best to just begin with some simple tools, try them out, and adjust as necessary.

Before we drop the mic on this chapter and move on, I want to touch on one more concept that I think is super useful here, and it's one of the reasons why the Four *R*s work so well. It's because in and of themselves, they're countering some of our brain's essential wiring to focus on the negative.

BATTLING NEGATIVITY BIAS

Perhaps you've heard about *negativity bias.* It's our brain's tendency to focus on the negative over the positive. Like, how four really good things could happen in your day, but you'll zero in on the one bad thing. Yes, you got a sweet card from your bestie in the mail, your hair is doing that thing you love, your boss really liked your work on that project, the deli down the street has your favorite special today . . . but then you spilled some lentil soup on your shirt at lunch. *DAMNIT! Why, God, whyyyy? Why does EVERYTHING have to go wrong?*

It's kind of a bummer that for most of us, our brains have a natural tendency to favor negative stimuli over positive. It makes it easier to dwell on things we perceive as bad and tougher to move past them. It can seem kind of shitty that we're like this—like our brains are betraying us. But here's a more positive take: this might be a default setting, but we can change it. Granted, it's not as easy as, say, swiping the toggle on your phone to switch to night mode, but it's totally possible. That's because another thing our brains are really good at is making things we repeat—thoughts, behaviors, and so on—easier to keep repeating.

Over time and with some practice engaging the *R*s, they will become easier to keep engaging. They'll become more automatic, and that's what we want. So, while it might feel like an uphill battle at first, remember that it's kind of like getting off the mental couch and expecting to run a marathon. For it to get easier, you gotta train, and that also counts for your brain. You got me? So even if you struggle at first, which is totally normal and I totally did as well, *it will get better.*

I want to take a second, too, to tag this chapter as one you'll probably want to revisit periodically, reminding yourself of the basics. As you sail along, sometimes you'll lose your bearings. Again, that's totally natural. That's why it's good to have this chapter on speed dial, so you can reread it and remind yourself of these concepts and tools as needed.

Now, onward! The next chapter is all about engaging a mindset of healing and learning how to truly be in recovery mode. Next stop: Safe Harbor.

EIGHT

CREATING SPACE FOR HEALING

When I was a kid, I was a vivacious, joyous little girl crackling with creative spirit. For as long as I can remember, I loved performing. From dancing and singing to plays, I *lived* for the stage. I have a photo of myself as a teeny tiny peanut with my neck bent all the way back, staring up at the TV screen watching Stephen Sondheim's musical *Into the Woods*. All of it was just so magical.

Even from that early age, I had a clear idea of who I wanted to be in the world: an actor. That's it. No question. And I built my whole identity around that ambition.

After high school I was accepted into a college with a wonderful theater department—Syracuse University—where I received my BFA. After graduation I returned to New York, auditioned, and booked jobs. I was lit up because by all accounts, my dream was starting to come true. Eventually I decided I would move to LA and focus on film, as my teachers had always suggested.

I was getting ready to do just that when *BAM!* I got sick. Almost overnight everything I knew to be true about myself shifted radically. I was twenty-five years old and went from having my whole future in front of me, one where everything was possible, to being so ill I could barely eat or walk more than a few steps (much less sing and dance). Suddenly this once-vibrant person was stuck in the hospital, trying desperately not to scratch the hives that covered my body and hooked up to an IV for the nourishment I needed to retain the most basic level of function.

When I first got sick, my doctor at the time sent me to a center for IV treatment. I'd sit there in a sticky gray plastic reclining chair with a frilly pillow (an afterthought if ever there was one) as medicine was infused into my veins. I would sit for hours waiting for the drip, drip, drip to finish, then wait even longer to let it all settle in. Then I'd have to go home and rest because the entire thing was so exhausting and the meds left me feeling completely wiped out.

This went on in one form or another for ten unhappy years—from a million tests to vitamin B12 injections to intravenous detox therapies. They were basically just throwing things at the wall to see what would stick. In the process, my life became about one thing: survival. I was just trying to make it through.

Eventually, of course, I got the right diagnosis and began to actually, fully heal. As part of that process, I got some routine bloodwork and my doctor noticed that my iron levels were low, so he suggested I get an IV infusion. Wouldn't you know I ended up back at the same center where I'd spent so much time before as a professional patient.

A new nurse practitioner was there and hooked me up to the first of two IVs. I could feel her nerves as I walked in. As we chatted, she said, "You're one of my first patients! I read your chart, and I was nervous about what kind of shape you were going to be in. The last time you were here, you were so, so sick! I thought you were going to come in such a mess today. I'm so happy to see you look so strong now. Way better than what I was expecting."

Have you ever had one of those moments where someone mirrors something back to you that you were totally unaware of? It's shocking, right? I had to sit there and let her words sink in. Because the thing was, in all that inching forward I'd done over the previous ten years, I'd never actually stopped to look back and see how far I'd come, or to truly digest what I'd been through. Out of curiosity, I asked her to tell me what she'd read in my file. And she did. And it took her so long to list out all the notes that by the time she was done, the IV bag was nearly empty.

Truth be told, it took a while to process what she'd said, in part because I felt so conflicted. On one hand there was this deep sense of sadness for my younger self, but also gratitude and relief at feeling like I was actually on the other side of it—at least for the most part. But mostly it was sadness. In my mind I pictured myself sitting in the same room, wearing my giant headphones, listening to Beyoncé, overwhelmed by all the effing *F*s, terrified, having eight thousand symptoms and no answers, receiving treatment for a diagnosis that turned out not to be true, desperately trying to just keep functioning. I had never seen it so clearly as I did in that moment, and my heart broke into a million pieces.

Then I remembered that from that enormous list, I was down to only three diagnoses: tick infections, hypothyroidism, and GI issues. I felt a surge of relief and thankfulness for how far I'd come. But that former me was lodged in my heart. It was only when I was emerging from a constant state of being in fight-or-flight mode that I could truly see that past version of me and start feeling the feels that came with it. And boy, did I do some feeling.

It all started to sink in. How my entire life—my dreams and plans and my big move to LA—had been put on hold. I was like a show that had been put on a sudden, indefinite hiatus. But now what?

A few weeks later, I went to the gym to work out (something I couldn't have even imagined doing a few years before that). I had a class with a trainer I'd never met before. She was young, blonde, and had this combination of strength and breeziness about her.

After we finished, we started chatting. It turned out we'd both gone to the same school and that she had studied musical theater. She was so vibrant and passionate about art. *What a breath of fresh air,* I thought. Then it struck me: *It's like I was talking to myself fifteen years ago!*

Then her next client showed up. As I turned to leave, she called after me, "Have you done anything with it?"

I froze mid-stride, my back still toward her. I felt my spirit sink into my shoes. I tried to get out of there, doing that nervous blurting, kind of half-turned toward her but still walking. "Uh, I did for a while. I trained in film and had a plan to move to LA, and then, well I got sick. Like really, really sick. And then my whole life kind of became about that."

She looked at me inquisitively, clearly sorry for what had happened, but she didn't say anything. It was the same kind of long pause I'd experienced so many times before when sharing my story. I broke the silence and told her about writing *Kicking Sick* but added that I missed performing. "Well," she said, "why don't you get back into it?"

I didn't know what to say. There I was, sweaty in my gym clothes, suddenly hurled back into thinking about this whole other life I'd had, and the loss of that future. "I'll think about it," I said, then tossed her a smile and headed out the door.

For the next few days, the episode played on repeat in my brain.

Following so close on the IV experience, it was like I'd just dropped down into a deeper layer of realization, seeing so clearly how much of my life had slipped out of my grasp. It was like I'd gone through a terrible time machine that spit me out fourteen years into the future. Now, here I was, a thirty-nine-year-old woman going through my life as if nothing had happened, and yet everything had happened, and everything had changed.

The next weekend Danny and I had tickets to a Broadway show I had been waiting to see for over a year—a revival of *Merrily We Roll Along.* I was so excited. Then, during the second half of the performance, Daniel Radcliffe began to sing the lyrics from "Good Thing Going," the song I'd used to audition for college. CLUNK. The bottom dropped even lower.

Sitting in that theater, I was overcome.

Where did my life go?!

It wasn't just heartbreaking, it was disorienting. There I was, thinking I had finally gotten to the other side of something. But I wasn't on the other side. Physically, yes, I was feeling a ton better. But mentally and emotionally I was somewhere in the middle, stuck in a kind of limbo. And I had no idea what to do, or where to go from there. It was a truth I wasn't prepared for, one that landed waaaay down inside me with a resounding thud.

But, how about you? I'm curious whether any of that sounds familiar to you, and I'm betting the answer is a big old Y-E-S. Have you ever been doing something you're so focused on, you look up at the clock and can't believe how much time has gone by? *How did it get to be four o'clock already?!* Well, for people with chronic illness, whole chunks of our life are like that. We're so zoomed in on our health and trying to heal that almost everything else becomes peripheral. Then one day we look up, and it's like, *How did I get to be forty already?!* I was twenty-five and then I blinked.

THE BIZARRE TIME WARP OF HEALING

Here's the thing: Remember in chapter 5 when we talked about the lack of a plan? How so often, the Western medical system treats you in the acute stage, then you're essentially dumped out on the curb? Well, this is the mental-emotional aspect of that. You go through this huge, long episode (or series of episodes), and all you're trying to do during that time is just that—get through it. Then *POP!* There you are, somewhere else. But . . . where?

Because it's not like you can just pick up where you left off from life. While you were so busy surviving, life went on. People around you changed. Your life stage changed. The place where you left off? Well, it might not even exist anymore.

About a year ago I was sitting on the couch, assuming the position for my weekly dose of the TV show *This Is Us*, which is a real emotion-fest in the best way. But what was usually a little sniffle for me surged into a full-blown snotty, can't breathe, ugly cry.

You see, in this particular episode, the matriarch of the show was at the end of her life, and all of her kids and grandkids had come to visit her to say goodbye. (Take it easy! No spoilers here.) Now, let's be clear guys, I am a proud cryer. I love a good cry. I think everyone should have a good cry often. No shame in my game on this one. However, what began as a normal cry became one of the most unexpected guttural sobs I have ever experienced. I wasn't sure what to make of the explosion of deep grief that had suddenly come over me, but I didn't think too much about it. After that night, though, I felt as tender as a Care Bear's belly, with a nose stuffed so completely I was mouth breathing for A DAY.

In the days that followed, I started to piece things together, and as I did it dawned on me how much I had compartmentalized the idea of motherhood. I am a very nurturing person by nature, and I love children. I had always wanted kids. When I was younger it was never a question whether or not I wanted to have a family. As far as I saw it, it was a given.

However, my life circumstances had put me on an entirely different path—one I wasn't prepared for. The rug had been ripped out from under me, and for close to fifteen years I was on the survival stress roller-coaster. As this was happening, periodically I'd think about starting a family and think, *It's just not the right time.* Then later, *Maybe it's not for me. It might not be in the cards.* But I never really processed that idea. I think in the back of my mind that when it came time to make a decision, there would still be a decision to be made. That having a family would still be an option.

But there I was on my bathroom floor, exhausted and vulnerable, having an internal crisis. *I was twenty-five, and now I am forty. I might not want to miss this moment. But what if I've already missed it? What if it's too late? And what would that even look like for me? How would my body even handle carrying a child? Do I want to stress my body further to do this? And does Lyme carry in utero?*

In the space of a TV episode I'd gone from this place where I still had time to feeling like I was up against the wall. In the end, I realized that the sadness I felt wasn't as much about me wanting to have a child and feeling pulled about it; it was more about missing the window in which I had the space and the ability to make a thoughtful choice about it. The option of kids had felt totally unattainable for so incredibly long; I had just stuffed it away in my mind, because in the moment, I couldn't see, feel, or deal. On my couch that night, my MTB now tamed, there it was, pounding on my front door.

When your health is no longer the central focus of your every waking moment, you have to pause for a minute so the world can stop spinning. To assess where your life is and figure out what you can pick back up again, and what you can't. Still, it feels like you're supposed to just jump back in, like hopping on a moving treadmill.

Remember my friend Lori who talked about how she felt like she was more than a decade behind her peers when it came to her career? There she was, trying to put her life back together and recover her health, and on top of it she felt like she was playing a giant game of catch-up.

Sitting in that theater watching *Merrily We Roll Along*, I was overwhelmed with a mixture of sadness and grief. That younger version of me had such a bright future but it's like her life was cut short. Instead, I was catapulted into a different world. It was like a *Sliding Doors* moment. In that movie we see two versions of a potential future for the main character, Helen. And it all boils down to whether or not she makes it onto a single train, or whether the doors close before she can hop on. The version of her who makes it leads one life, while the one left standing on the platform takes an entirely different path.

The thing I had yet to realize, that would sink in over the next days, weeks, and months, was that I hadn't shifted to an alternate universe. *This was still my life*. It felt like it had been split in two, and Young Actor Amy had become Older, Formerly Sick Amy. Life before illness, and life after illness. One where I had everything I wanted at the time, and one where everything had been taken from me. But, as I'd come to understand, that wasn't the case. It was still one life—my life—but it was in progress. In the middle. And to end up on the other side, I needed time and space to heal. And I needed to create that for myself. I needed the chance to catch my breath and to understand that even if the train I expected to take had left the station, there is always another one pulling in shortly.

And you need that time and space for yourself, too. Because when we try to just jump back in? It's totally disorienting, and that's because we're skipping a step: the space where we recover. Where we heal, recalibrate, and reorient. We need time to let the snow globe settle. That space actually already has a name: convalescence. And it's a space no one else can give you. You have to create it for yourself.

CONVALESCENCE: NOT JUST FOR GRANDMAS

If you're like I was not so long ago, the word *convalescence* conjured some fairly antiquated or just old-adjacent images. As in, "How's grandma doing after her hip surgery?" "Oh, pretty good—they just transferred her to the convalescent home." Then there's that season of *Downton Abbey* where they transformed part of the mansion into a convalescent home for World War I officers. That kind of thing. Personally I've struggled with the word because it sounds so, well, geriatric. Like, if convalescence was a perfume, its smell would be somewhere between moth balls, potpourri, and makeup powder.

The word *rehab* doesn't really work because it's the territory of twelve-step programs. Same with *recovery. Mending?* Meh. Sounds like something you do after a breakup, or like fixing a hole in a sock. *Revival?* That happens in church. So, convalescence it is! I'm gonna learn to like that word, I swear. I bet you will, too.

Convalescence is really just a recovery period after a major illness or injury.

A what, now?

Say it with me out loud: RECOVERY PERIOD.

It's wild, because if you go through chemo or rotator cuff surgery, it's a given that you'll need some kind of after care, but not so with chronic illness. It's like, they just don't get how deeply we're affected.

Recently I went to try biomagnetic therapy. A few of my friends have had really good results with it, so I figured I'd check it out. At one point the doctor was chatting with me, describing something or other. He said, yadda yadda yadda, "that mostly pertains to someone with severe stress, like loss of a job, or folding of a company, or divorce. Not stuff like this." *Stuff like this,* meaning chronic illness and the associated trauma.

I smiled and counted to three, then said, "Okay, so what about having the rug ripped out from under you by getting sick, and life as you know it shifting on a dime in every way? Does that count?" Wink wink, nudge nudge.

He gave me one of those uncomfortable laughs and said, "Well . . . yes. I suppose it does."

We both kept a good attitude about it and shared a chuckle, but I mean seriously? He was saying the quiet part out loud, admitting the lack of understanding that I think so many providers have about what we really go through and how it *affects* us.

But not here, my dear. I get what you've been through and where you are, and I know that it takes real time and effort to heal. Yes, effort. Here's the thing: Convalescence isn't just about rest. That can be an important component, but it's so much more than that. It's about creating a healing space where you can catch up with yourself and start to truly process all that you've been through. You've got to really engage with the process.

I know what you might be thinking: *But I can't take more time off! I have to get back to work/parenting/relationships. I don't have a Victorian estate to go back to and lay on a chaise longue in sensory deprivation with only candlelight,* etc. . . . I hear you! The good news is that even if you don't have the luxury of an actual break from life—which most of us don't—you can still convalesce. In a minute, I'll show you how. But for now, we're going to get clear on convalescence as a concept: what it entails, and how it can help us heal.

One of the key concepts of convalescence is self-care. But, it might not be self-care as you typically think of it. This is particularly important for all the gals out there, but at its heart it applies to everyone. So often, it's difficult for us as women to put our needs first and to spend so much time (or really, any time at all) caring for ourselves. Somehow it feels . . . *unnatural.* There are a few reasons for that.

For one, there's the long-time cultural expectation that women are meant to give and give endlessly, without regard for ourselves. In so many spaces that behavior is encouraged and even celebrated. (How many times have you heard a woman praised for being "selfless"?) But beyond that there's also biology. We have that deep caregiver wiring. (Not that men don't have this, but biologically speaking it's different for women.)

The upshot is that we might feel reluctant to devote time to ourselves. Maybe it feels selfish or wrong. Or perhaps it feels like a weakness. In a culture that prizes success and productivity, all of us (of every gender) are under pressure to do, do, DO! It's the same whether you're working, parenting, or in any sphere. Your value is in what you produce, and if you're not giving your maximum, there's something wrong with you.

What it comes down to is that focusing on yourself might feel really hard to do, at least at first. But as with so many things it will get easier, we've just gotta take those baby steps. And speaking of babies . . .

We all get how babies need extra care, right? Well, we sort of need to be in that mode with ourselves right now. To see ourselves as more tender, vulnerable versions of ourselves who need that extra attention and care at this point in our lives. Maybe see yourself as a younger version of you, if that helps. I actually have a photo of lil' Amy on my phone that I pull up every time I'm feeling run down, upset, or like I haven't been listening to myself. Looking at that picture reminds me that little me is still inside, and she still needs my loving attention.

Recovery mode is about being gentle with yourself. Think about an athlete who's recovering from an injury. They're not out there going hard, trying to set a record. They're taking the time to heal. They're doing sauna, getting massages, eating all the healthy food, maximizing sleep. They're rocking those bad-ass cupping marks. Basically, they're pouring every bit of energy they can into caring for themselves, and we totally respect them for that! But when it comes to us, we can have a really hard time doing the equivalent. Instead, we might see ourselves as slackers and think we should just be able to get back in the game already!

But if you think about it, no one looks at an injured athlete who's taking time off and is like, "Lightweight!" We understand that not caring for an injury is likely to delay healing or make things worse. The same is true for us! Remember that what you're recovering from is a *psychic injury*. And if you want to experience that post-traumatic growth we talked about, that comes down to giving yourself actual time and space to heal.

If I accomplish one thing in this chapter, please let it be that you come out the other side understanding that caring for yourself is a *strength*, not a weakness.

Self-care is not a bubble bath, or a manicure, or a massage. Sure, it can include those things if that's helpful for you, and I say this as someone who is a tried-and-true lover of a bath. But *self-care is not a luxury*! It's not a treat. And it's not self-indulgent. And we need to stop thinking about it like it is, especially when we're trying to heal. Self-care is *essential.* It's mandatory, and it's make-or-break.

At the most fundamental level, there is care that you can only give yourself. Grace, compassion, love, patience—it's wonderful to receive these from others, but it's most important that you give them to yourself. And, whenever possible, to prioritize it above all other things!

Now, I'm going to add a carve-out here for parents and other caregivers. There are times in life when we technically have to put others first because they can't care for themselves. As my friend Kira pointed out, that can be an extremely difficult balancing act, because it can feel like if you're doing something for yourself, you're taking away from them.

Sometimes, other people do come first. The problem is when this becomes our default mode, and we lose sight of just how critically we need care ourselves. So I'm encouraging you, especially at this time, to put yourself first *whenever you can.* That's part of the mindset of convalescence. In this space, you at least get to be me-first more often. You have to do that if you want to heal. And kids are more likely to thrive when they have healthy parents, got it?

If you're pressed for opportunities to do that, you might need to schedule time for yourself. Write it on your calendar. Schedule time for rest, for walks, for feeling your feelings.

Plus, if you parents need extra convincing, remember this: When you care for yourself, you're modeling that for your kids! Otherwise, they might look at you and think that being a parent means always putting yourself last and looking (and feeling) like a dishrag. And they might ingest the idea that we should always just push through. That's probably not a message you intend to send.

Are we clear? Good!

Now I want to pivot and talk about something that's really central to convalescence and allowing space for healing, and that's learning to welcome and work with grief.

GOOD GRIEF

In part one, we mentioned briefly the idea of grief. Now, it's time to dig in. But wait, why now, exactly? Well, for two reasons. The first is that when we finally slow down and give ourselves space to heal, that might be the first time that our feelings actually catch up with us. It might be the first time we're actually aware of our grief and take account of the things we've lost. The second is that it's kind of a positive cycle: Convalescence allows grief the space to show up, and doing the work of grieving gives us the space to heal.

I had the opportunity to speak with Dr. Gina Moffa, a grief therapist and author of *Moving on Doesn't Mean Letting Go: A Modern Guide to Navigating Loss.* As she explains, grief is a natural element of the healing process. When our nervous system begins to thaw, and we start to shift out of constant survival mode, it's natural for emotions such as grief to rush in. And that's what happened to me. Maybe you're experiencing that, too. Have you ever had that experience where you're actually starting to feel better, like, *Hey, I'm having a good day today!* and then suddenly you're hit with all of these heavy emotions? It's like *POW*, where did that come from?

The thing about grief is that while it may not *feel* good, it *does* good. That is, if we can learn to work with it instead of against it. If we can allow grief to work its magic.

As Dr. Moffa explained, when we first experience a sense of loss, it puts us in a space where we don't have access to our inner resources. "Our nervous system feels like we're being attacked in some way," she says. "Any kind of loss we go through—whether it's a friendship loss, a pet loss, a job loss—will still affect the same part of the brain as losing a spouse." In other words, the way our nervous system metabolizes loss and the way it lights up our brain can be really similar regardless of whether you lost a loved one or part of your life. Let that land.

As Dr. Moffa describes it, our nervous system only speaks one language: safety and unsafety. That's why grief can launch us back into that survival, fight-or-flight mode where we can feel "untethered, unsafe, disconnected, and like you're waiting for the other shoe to drop." (I swear I didn't prompt the shoe thing. She said it on her own!)

I had the opportunity to interview Dr. Peter Levine, and he explained that when our nervous system starts to thaw out of a freeze state, where we might feel numb or disconnected, it's possible that we can ping into fight-or-flight mode, where we feel hyperalert. We can go from being tuned out to being tuned way-the-heck in, and that can be overwhelming. Suddenly there are all of these *feelings* and it's hard to manage them all. In the last chapter, I introduced you to some techniques to try when you feel flooded in this way, and we'll explore some more later on in the book.

For now, something I think is helpful to keep in mind is that *nothing is wrong with you*. This is actually part of the healing process, even if it feels confusing or disorienting or overwhelming. It's natural. It actually means that your nervous system is gaining capacity—which is what you want! It's just that the capacity is making space for all those feels to come rushing in. Including grief. And even though grief doesn't feel great, it does offer us a chance to do some pretty incredible things.

And the way I see it, there's also beauty to loss and grief. For one, this whole recovery process offers a chance to process not just what happened to you during your illness but also what's happened to you in life. Because there's a funny thing that happens when we grieve. We might be launched into grief by a specific loss, but then other losses we've experienced tend to piggyback on it. It's like, you're mourning the fact that you've lost entire parts of your life, and then suddenly you're thinking about your parents' divorce when you were eight, or the death of your childhood rabbit, Mr. Hoppers. He had those big fuzzy ears!!

That can feel overwhelming and like a bit of a WTF. But the positive of it is that you're in a space where you have this tremendous opportunity to work through all this shit you've been ignoring or were just unaware of. Stuff that's been piling up inside you. That's just one of the gifts of grief. And as it turns out, there are many.

In her beautiful book, *I'm Not a Mourning Person*, Kris Carr writes about how, "Grief cracks you open and teaches you priceless, heart expanding, and healing lessons. . . . It can be used as a catalyst to take inventory of your life, figure out what matters most versus what you can let go of, and allow you to reset, breathing into the next phase of brave, courageous, and utterly unique *you*."

When I first read that it got me thinking: Isn't grief the loss of *everything* important in your life? This was at the time when I was just starting to process all that I'd lost. I was quiet for a few days. And then, do you know what I let myself do? Be a puddle. I cried and I let myself feel all my feelings (and, boy, were there plenty of them). Because sometimes we need to be brave enough to give ourselves permission to fall apart, to feel our feelings fully even when they seem unbearable.

In the Jewish tradition, after someone dies, their loved ones sit shiva. It's a time that provides spiritual and emotional healing as mourners gather to support each other. I sat shiva by myself and for myself. I mourned for the life that could have been, for the sparkly little girl inside me who had never gotten to realize her dreams, and for the pain of what I had gone through desperately seeking an answer to my health crisis.

And you know, I want to call out another aspect of sitting shiva that highlights one more of grief's gifts. It's that, when we let it, grief can actually fuel connection.

Scientists like to talk about things like why, evolutionarily, we feel certain things. How different feelings have helped us adapt and evolve. When you look at something like grief, you might think, *How on earth could that help to keep us alive?* One answer is: connection.

For one, loss is something that every single one of us will experience in life, and sharing it can help us feel more in tune with one another. I mean, just talking about grief and chronic illness, I feel more deeply connected to you, *and I can't even see you!* But I feel you and your heart. Hi, friend.

Connection and a sense of belonging are essential in life. And when we feel emotions like sadness and despair around loss, those things are actually encouraging us to reach out and touch someone. But as Dr. Mary-Francis O'Connor, psychologist and author of *The Grieving Brain*, explains, having help in grief isn't just a good thing, it's a *necessity*. As she says, "Grief is a universal experience, and when we can connect, it is better."

When you're grieving—similar to having a chronic illness in general—there's a point where society expects you to move on. To be done already! Maybe we expect that of ourselves, too. As Dr. Moffa told me: "Grief takes endurance. It's a really important thing to remember because it's so exhausting . . . and it can feel like it's never going to leave you." She calls this experience the middle phase of grief—meaning the phase that settles in after the initial awareness. And this is the part that requires the most presence and patience, because it's in this phase that we can start to feel like we're sinking. Dr. Moffa explains that's "because you're so busy trying to be what society wants you to be, which is normal and unaffected, and yet your whole world has changed. It's as if you're a brand new child in a brand new world. You're navigating a totally new landscape."

And this phase is also where you start to experience *secondary losses*. This includes the loss of money or a job from having been sick so long, maybe having to move because you can no longer afford your home. It can also look like an awareness of losing a role in life or a sense of purpose or identity (*ding!*).

In my conversation with Dr. Moffa, I brought up the idea of identity loss, and I shared my experience with her. I told her how I'd studied acting, then my sudden realization so many years later that I'd been forced off that train before my stop. And it felt like I'd lost a huge piece of myself. Yet Dr. Moffa challenged me on that notion. As it turned out, for different reasons, she'd had a similar experience, where she was certain she was going to do one thing but was forced to change tracks. She shared that if she constantly looked back at that other life and characterized it as the one she should have had, her current life would feel like a letdown. And it isn't.

In that conversation I realized something: I hadn't lost my identity. It wasn't *gone*. It had just, changed. And my story isn't over. I have no idea what the next chapter will be, but that's kind of the point. I don't know what it won't be either. What I mean is, I love my life. And I don't know what's in store. Is something I once loved gone forever, or is it maybe not? Or will the essence of what I loved about acting be alive in my life again someday, but maybe in a different way? I can honestly say that the process of healing has awakened some wonderful and powerful things in me. Things I am grateful for. I became a writer, and I channeled my creative energy from acting into this, and if I never did that, there wouldn't be you and me.

If you're struggling with a sense of identity loss or confusion, you can ask yourself questions like the ones I asked myself:

- What role or identity do I feel I've lost? (You might have more than one.)
- When I picture myself in that role or identity, what do I feel?
- What aspects or actions of the identity or role are most important to me?
- What are some other ways I can potentially express those aspects or essences?
- What are some other ways I can potentially experience those same or similar feelings?
- Are there any ways in which my identity has shifted for the better with this new perspective?

Since these questions are pretty deep, I encourage you to be patient—the answers might need some time to unfold. Writing about them in a journal or talking through them with a good friend could help.

This isn't about putting a happy face on something painful. Instead, it's about letting multiple things be true. You lost something and it feels painful. AND you are grateful for what you have now—or aspects of it—that you wouldn't otherwise.

As Dr. Maté put it when we spoke, the process of healing from MTB "is actually an opportunity for people to ask a lot of questions that they weren't in a position to ask before. Because they weren't in a position to answer them." And while those answers aren't always easy, each one forms a step on the path to healing.

I'm not trying to tell you how to relate to identity loss. Remember that we're taking our power back, people! That includes choosing how you view yourself and your experiences. You get to take agency over how you relate to your identity. I'm just sharing what has helped me. And that brings me back to the *Sliding Doors* idea because like I said, in the end, everything was okay. Both versions of Helen landed somewhere positive. So who's to say what was the right or wrong, good or bad, path? And who is to say that this isn't still your life just as much as it was before? It's another one of those ambiguous spaces, which again, can feel so disorienting and leave us feeling so disconnected.

As grief counselor Seanna Crosbie writes, "What makes secondary losses challenging is their often intangible nature, making it difficult for others to grasp the depth of their impact. This lack of visibility can lead to a diminishing support system over time, leaving you grappling with the hidden effects of loss."

The hardest phase of grief can also be the hardest part for others to understand the full breadth and depth of what you're going through. Yet it's also where you need the most support. Have you ever experienced a time when you're at your lowest and you need others most, but that's when you feel the least connected? Like the people around you just don't get what you're going through? It's seriously tough stuff.

This pile on can make you start to feel hopeless—like there's just too much for you to handle. Or you might start to feel anger, even rage, over all you've experienced. That can be scary, but it's totally normal. It can be tough to hang out with big feelings, so it can be best to take it in small bites.

The point is, sometimes we actually start to feel worse before we feel better, and that's part of the process. The same is true physically, because we don't just experience grief and other emotions in our brains; we also experience them in our body. You might have new symptoms you never had before, like brain fog, appetite loss, or sleep disruptions. As Irene Lyon told me, when you start the journey of healing trauma, it's really common to have points where you feel worse before you feel better, and this is why. Try to keep in mind that the upside of this is that the reason you're having these new feelings and body experiences is actually because things are changing inside you. Those changes can cause other shifts. When one symptom resolves another might arise, but try not to get discouraged because it can actually be signaling that you're on the right track. When your nervous system starts to gain more capacity to feel, well, more feelings show up. That's normal. And all of that can start to feel discouraging, to say the least, which is why connection is so important.

As Dr. Moffa told me: "When you're in a place where you feel like you're circling a drain and may drown . . . to do that alone puts us in a space of isolation. My hope is that everyone has at least one person who sees them and validates that their grief is still alive and present when society has already moved forward." Because without that, we can start to cave in on ourselves and become isolated. When we feel cut off from others, that's where grief can get artificially prolonged and turn into a mental health problem.

"It's about someone witnessing you and being a safe place," she said. Otherwise, that isolation can land you back in fight-flight-freeze mode. That's because your nervous system is like a smoke detector, always scanning for potential threats. But when you're with someone you trust or otherwise in a safe space, the smoke alarm gives the all clear. That lets your body *relax*. But no safe space, no relaxation. And no relaxation means no healing. And that's true at a cellular level.

Dr. Maté also called out the dangers of isolation, and he linked it to the loneliness and grief we feel when we can't be ourselves. As I've experienced it, throughout the course of our treatment, we have to put on masks to feel like we'll get the care we need. But that mask wearing creates a loss: the loss of identity. And those losses are exactly what hit me so hard when I got those one-two-three punches I described at the start of the chapter.

On the other hand, being witnessed, validated, and honored helps to put us in a healing zone. And that's part of what we're jump-starting in our convalescence—that process of being, and being seen for, who we really are.

Now, all of that might have felt like a real crash course on grief. I encourage you to sit with what you've read, and if it feels helpful, go back and read it again. Revisit, reflect, and digest. And grab a cozy chair, some fluffy slippers, because we're going to be in convalescence mode for a while.

Some aspects of healing are about connecting with other people, or at least one other person. But sometimes it's about deepening our connection with ourselves. And that's something that's essential to true healing.

To kick off the how-tos of recovery mode, let's start by creating a welcome space in your inner landscape. A place where you can chill out with the most important person in your recovery process: you.

MAKING CONVALESCENCE COOL AGAIN: HOW TO HEAL

Picture it: You're sitting on a big front porch overlooking a forest woodland, listening to the sounds of a stream trickling by. You're leaning back in a rocking chair, blanket in your lap, a steaming cup of tea on the table beside you.

Or perhaps you're lounging on the couch in a seaside cottage. The windows are open and you smell the salt air. You're lying there, eyes closed, listening to the sounds of seagulls with waves crashing in the distance.

Sounds nice, huh? The beauty of these scenes, or whatever relaxing getaway you fancy, is that even if we can't go there in reality, we can be there in our brains. It's like going to our mental happy place.

And that's actually the crux of convalescence: more than anything you do, it's a state of mind. Think of it like creating an Airbnb inside you, and no matter what's going on in the outside world, it's a peaceful space you can visit as you recover.

I'm fully aware that idea might sound a little hokey, but really, it's just a form of visualization. Having a mental happy place—or at least a peaceful one—is a way of bringing some calm into your world. Here's a visualization to help you get started building your happy place:

1. Get into a comfortable position—maybe it's seated in a chair, maybe it's laying on the floor, maybe it's in a bubble bath.
2. If you feel ready, close your eyes.
3. Take a deep breath in to the count of three, pause, then out to the count of three. Repeat that breathing pattern through this visualization.
4. Now, imagine you're in a place that makes you feel calm, relaxed, supported, and safe. It could be an actual place you've been in the past, or a place entirely of your imagining.
5. What do you see around you? Is there an ocean? Mountains? Framed photos of your family on the wall? Some animal besties?
6. Now, what do you hear? Ocean waves lapping, wind rustling through leaves? Birdsong? Some gentle piano music?

7. And what do you smell? Fresh sagebrush after a rain? Your favorite stew simmering on the stove? The soft smoke of a campfire?
8. Hang out in your happy place. Take in the details. What else do your senses reveal?
9. When you're ready, take one more nice, long inhale, then slowly exhale and open your eyes.
10. Take a moment to gently stretch, roll your shoulders, turn your head side to side.

The great news is that your happy place is open 24/7, and it's totally free! Go there any time you need a short getaway. I am not just telling you to do this, friends. I'm walking the talk. My happy place is Turks and Caicos, sitting with my feet in the white clay sand, watching the sunset-tinted water crash into tiny waves. Because as you're doing the work of re-regulating your nervous system, you could certainly use a bit of that. And something you'll need *a lot* of is self-care.

BUILDING BOUNDARIES: THE HEALING BUBBLE

There's a lot of great material out there about the importance of boundaries and being able to say no. Again, this is something that women, especially, can feel challenged to do. Societally we're expected to be givers. Here again, though, it's not an option. When you're in recovery mode, you need that extra time and energy to direct toward your healing. If you're expecting yourself to show up for everyone else, you don't have the capacity to process your experience or your feelings.

For me, when I'm in convalescence mode, I enact a personal policy. I only say yes to people and events that make me feel energized. If something's likely to be a downer or leave me feeling drained, it's a hard no. Granted, sometimes I make exceptions, but I try to be really thoughtful about them, and to make them rare.

That's because I think about events or people or surroundings not just physically, like how my body will feel, but also energetically. We've talked about the importance of connection, but it's also important to protect our own energy. Any time you're interacting with someone is an energetic exchange. Have you ever noticed that if you're hanging out with someone who is especially anxious or negative, you also start to feel a little on edge? It's because you're picking up their energy. So, when I know that I'm going to places that will be physically draining, I try to keep a bubble around me. Inside is the totally safe space—I'm in my mental Airbnb—and the rest of the world and all its attitudes, opinions, judgments, and pressures are locked outside.

It's not about shutting people out, per se, but about being really selective about who you allow to be close to you, especially at those times when you're feeling particularly vulnerable. There are times when Danny's the only one who gets to be in my inner circle, and everyone else is relegated to the outer realms. It's not personal, it's just what I need.

If you have people in your life who can be exhausting or judgmental or insensitive or any of those other negative things humans can be, to the extent that you can, I encourage you to keep your distance. At least when you're at your most vulnerable.

If your immune system was challenged, you wouldn't lick a door handle. (Okay, I hope you'd never actually lick a door handle, but work with me for a minute.) Think of this as a time when your mental-emotional immune system is low, and those folks are contagious. You do not need to be exposed to or infected with their negativity. This is a time when only supportive people get to be close. And if anyone argues with you, tell 'em I said so!

If you do have to engage with people or situations that will likely leave you drained, I like doing this protective visualization/meditation. Imagining that there's a protective layer around me helps ensure that any of that negative energy won't seep in too deeply. Here's a visualization I find especially helpful.

1. Get in a comfortable position and take a few nice deep breaths and close your eyes if you feel okay doing so. Relax your shoulders, and take a moment to feel your feet contact the floor (or your heels if you're laying down).
2. Imagine a basic map of our solar system. Don't worry if you don't get the names and the orders of all the planets right. I rarely do.
3. Picture yourself as the sun, so you're looking out as all of these celestial bodies are orbiting you.
4. Now, imagine these planets are populated by the people in your life. You get to decide who goes where. Who is safe enough and feels good enough to be closer, on Mercury or Venus? Who needs to stay out on Neptune?
5. Let this image play in your mind for a bit, feeling the difference distances of each of these people from you.
6. Open your eyes. Now, when you actually interact with these people, picture the planet they're on and remind yourself that's as close as their energy can get to you.

But it's not just about people and spaces that feel negative. It can just be about the bandwidth that things require. Even if something feels like it would be fun—like going to a bachelorette weekend—it might just be too much. When you're in this healing space, you gotta be real with yourself about your resources. You gotta ask yourself: Will this contribute to or detract from my healing? This also counts for social media, too. Be thoughtful about the content you expose yourself to.

When it comes down to it, you're the only one who can make that call. And that's why it's imperative that you connect with yourself. To keep checking in, knowing that each day, hour, or even minute might be asking you for something different. So, it's essential to pay attention to what you need.

The big WOW of this is that this could be the first time in your life that you've actually done that. And that's another one of the gifts of grief and convalescence: They call us into ourselves. They call us home, if we listen closely to their whisper. And maybe it's the first time we've ever tuned into ourselves in that way. But once you do—once you learn to listen to your own frequency—you can start attending to yourself in deeper ways. And that's what helps you heal. Not just from MTB, but from all kinds of stuff you've experienced. And that? Well, it's kind of beautiful.

As we start to develop a deeper connection with ourselves, work through our grief, and heal, we start to gain our bearings again. We just have to have faith in ourselves that we can do it. Faith, patience, and a ton of self-love.

But of course, that's not all. There's also self-trust, and in the next chapter, we'll look at how to start rebuilding it.

NINE

NO MORE MASKS

Of all the things that happened to me in the ten-plus years I struggled intensively with chronic illness, the worst was losing my sense of self. Becoming disconnected from my identity was part of it, but it was more than that.

In virtually all of my interactions with the medical system, it was drilled into me, time and time again, that other people knew more about me and what was best for me than I did. Over time I learned to put my own ideas and intuition on mute, ignoring what they were telling me. I agreed to procedures, treatments, and tests that didn't feel right to me intuitively and that I didn't want. In short, I gave my power away.

To be crystal clear, if that sounds like I'm blaming myself, I'm not. I'm just owning it. With very few exceptions, all of the external forces in my world were encouraging me to, in essence, do what I was told and all would be fine. So I did. And when it comes to the medical system, I think most of us do that to some extent. But it wasn't fine. The choice to override my own authority had real consequences.

It's no coincidence that the doctor who finally got me a correct diagnosis(es) was also the first medical care provider to encourage me to own my role in my own health care. He didn't just want me to step up, he required it. But as I described in chapter 6 that was *so hard to do* at first. That's how little I trusted myself. Sound familiar to you?

Yet here's the good news. Though it took a lot of time and energy, I was able to baby step myself back into the right relationship with the person who truly does know me best. And as the people in my life will tell you, these days there are no *Yes, sir*s or *Yes, ma'ams* coming out of my mouth. I am right in there, involved in all the stuff, asking questions and making my thoughts and feelings known. And as I've found, that kind of engagement isn't just good for my physical healing, it's also been essential for my mental and emotional recovery.

The reality is, when you become that disconnected from yourself, it can be really hard to make your way back. To come home. But that's the good thing about a true home—it's always right there waiting for you. Your soul or spirit or the deepest part of you or whatever you want to call it? It's really patient, loves you unconditionally, and it doesn't hold grudges. So as far apart from your true self as you might feel right now, you haven't actually lost anything. It's still right there, with some soup on the stove and fresh flowers on the table, waiting for you.

REBUILDING TRUST

As with all of this healing stuff, rebuilding your relationship with yourself takes time. That's because all healing in one form or another happens at a cellular level, bit by bit. Healing trauma is not just about shifting your thoughts, it's about getting way down in there like an underground electrician and doing some rewiring; disconnecting this wire, plugging that one back in.

Just like so much we've talked about, the essential first step takes place at the level of the nervous system. Now, you've already started this work by engaging the kinds of tools and techniques we talked about in chapter 8. You've already opened the lines of conscious communication between you and your deeper self. Now, we're going to add a practice that's so simple it's kinda funny. But it works, and it's important to the process of rebuilding trust. And it all starts with peeing.

LISTENING TO YOUR BODY

Yeah, you read that right: I said *peeing*. But it's not just that, it's also drinking and eating and sleeping, too. All the basics. Here, I'll explain.

You can't just suddenly appear on the scene and tell your brain-body, "Okay, I'm back! I'm listening now! What's up?" and expect it to just respond. Let's say you had a good friend who was an amazing communicator. They'd call, text, send cards, but a lot of the time, for a long time, you just ignored them. So, their messages start to dwindle. But then one day you suddenly drop into their texts, "Hey, it's me! I'm so sorry I ignored you. But I'm back! Let's be besties." Crickets.

Understandably, your friend is probably going to be a little wary of just taking your word for it. So, what can you do? You have to *prove you're for real*. That means walking the talk. When your friend calls, you have to pick up! When they text you a funny gif, emoji them back. If they wanna hang out, make time for them. After a while, they'll start to trust you again, but you have to show you mean it.

Here's what that looks like in your body. You've spent a lot of time muting your body's signals. Like when you electively tried ten thousand supplements at once and had no idea what was causing you to feel bloated, but you just kept it all in the plan, ignoring your body's nudges. Or when the physician assistant dismissed the symptoms you shared as "unrelated" and you wanted to push back, but instead you bit your tongue. Or when you went to get bloodwork and the person couldn't find the vein, so you spent five pricks going against your instinct instead of being brave and asking for someone new. When we force down or ignore internal signals, especially when all of that is mixed in with survival stress, it becomes like a venti trauma Frappuccino with extra whip—ordered by no one ever.

The result is that it can take some convincing to get your brainbody to talk to you again. So how do you do that? Show your brainbody you are listening by responding to its most basic signals. For instance, when you're sitting there reading an incredible book (eh-hem) and your body signals, "I have to pee!" stop reading and go pee. Ditto for listening to drinking some water when you're thirsty, eating when it's mealtime, and going to bed when you're sleepy instead of staying up to binge season nineteen of *Sister Wives.*

This is how Irene Lyon described it to me when we spoke: Functions like digestion are governed by the "automatic" part of our nervous system (technically called the *autonomic* nervous system). "So if we're always holding in these responses or completely disconnected from them (which is most of the time, I find, because people have disconnected from their bodies because of trauma and not being able to feel and not being allowed to feel) they start losing what's called *interoception.* [It's that internal sensing that] lets us know *I gotta to pee, I'm tired, I'm thirsty, I'm cold, I don't feel so well, I think I'm coming down with something.* It gives us that cue: *I need to pay attention.*"

We ignore our bodies and our nervous systems all the time and think little of it. Either we don't pee when we have to—gotta get that email written!—or we don't drink when we're thirsty because we don't want to have to get up to pee. Or we don't sleep when we're legitimately tired because we'd rather watch TV. All of that sends a deep message about what we value and prioritize, and it isn't our own fundamental needs. It keeps us dysregulated and disconnected. But we can change that.

Lyon characterized it like this: "I kind of call it a reverse engineering in that as simple as it is, if an adult knows that they have dysregulation, and they're struggling, you start listening to those simple things, like when there's pressure in your bladder. Because the moment you relieve that, it sends feedback to your autonomic nervous system saying, 'Hey, we're listening to you.'" Over time, your interoception starts to come back online. It's like, suddenly you're tuned in to the same frequency that your body has been trying to broadcast all of these messages on, and they're finally coming through!

So that's step one: As much as you can (acknowledging that you can't always just veer off the highway the second you have to pee), make it a priority to notice and respond to your body's signals. Treat them like they're important, because they are. Over time, your body will start to send you all kinds of messages you weren't getting, or at least weren't noticing, before. It will feel like you're suddenly plugged into this magical source of information (because you are) or like your intuition is on overdrive. Think about it like this: Your body was screaming from the top of the mountain to get you to realize you were sick in the first place and you needed to pay attention. So, you did. Your body is brilliant—the very best expert on *you*—and it wants to send you signals. You just have to choose to tune in to its subtleties, and when you do, it's the most incredible and intimate relationship.

These days, I think of it as caring for my internal peanut. So when Little Amy taps me on the shoulder and whispers, "I'm tired. I don't wanna go out tonight," I listen. I mean, would you drag a sleepy kid in footie pajamas out to a party? Yet we do some version of that all the time, and it amounts to not listening to ourselves on a fundamental level. And when we do that a lot, we start to feel disconnected from ourselves, because in a very real way we are. If a kid comes to you over and over asking for things and you ignore them, after a while they stop asking. You have got to stop what you're doing and give them your attention and your care.

Granted, we can't always just drop everything we're doing or change all of our plans. Sometimes it's just not feasible to respond to every request, or at least do so right away. You just want to prioritize those deep needs as often as possible. It's really similar to what we talked about in the last chapter in terms of protecting your energy and seeing self-care as essential. These are overlapping circles on the same Venn diagram, and they all contribute to re-establishing your sense of self and rebuilding trust.

Here's something that's really cool: this idea of disconnection isn't only rooted in MTB. We can experience it for all kinds of reasons, and our environment supports and encourages it. I'm talking social media, video games, *The Real Housewives of Salt Lake City*... all the stuff that's designed to capture our attention and not let go. But with the messy trauma slurpy of MTB mixed all up in there, it can be even harder to reconnect. Yet you can, and it starts here. And when you do that work, the healing is exponential. Meaning, it goes beyond just healing MTB, but repairing those disconnects that happened for all kinds of other reasons. It's a massive win.

RE-MEETING YOURSELF

As your brain-body starts to re-engage with you more, it's normal to feel a little off-kilter. What I mean is, imagine that old friend again. While you know you still love and care about one another, you haven't really talked for a while, so when you finally start hanging out again, it might feel a little awkward at first. And it's easy to presume that they are the same person as when you last spoke. But the reality is, a lot has changed. And it has with you, too.

In our culture we are absolutely smitten with the phrase "back to normal." But I pretty much guarantee you that in nearly every case where this phrase is invoked, there is no such thing. (COVID, anyone?) Life, and the people in it, are constantly shifting, so in essence there's rarely something we can truly go back to. If we're always chasing the past, we'll never catch it, and that can leave us feeling like we've irrevocably lost something. In a sense, that's true. And in another sense, it's not. Again, it's one of those both/and situations.

Instead of normal being a place in the past, try thinking of it as the baseline you create in the moment. And that you recreate as circumstances change. In other words, it's time for (yes, I'm gonna say it) *a new normal.*

When it comes to your relationship with yourself, that means not expecting yourself to ever go back to being "the old you." Instead, you can be open to who you are now, in this moment. Of course you have aspects of yourself, your personality, and so on that have always been there and are still there now (my sarcasm and sense of caution run *deep*!). But you've also changed. You've been through a lot. You've got new perspectives, new strengths, new insights. So, your body-brain might have some surprising and unexpected things to communicate to you. Like, *I know you like that friend, but I don't know if she's good for you. I don't think she always has your best interests at heart, and I don't think you feel so good after hanging out with her.* Or, *I know you love peanut butter, but while eating a tub of it with a spoon might be both satisfying and delicious, I think it's causing those breakouts you keep having.*

This is where a practice like free writing can be super helpful. It's simple—you just sit down with a blank piece of paper (yes, this is more effective with actual handwriting rather than typing on a computer, but it's not essential) and let 'er rip. Write down whatever words or thoughts come to mind.

Often, it's helpful to have a prompt to get started. I like to pretend that I'm talking to the paper, so I'll start by asking myself something like:

- What would you like to tell me that you don't think I know?
- What am I missing when I look in the mirror?
- What's deeply true about me and who I am that I'm not seeing?
- And here's my favorite: What's the cost to me of putting on a mask, and is it worth it? What's the impact on my mental and emotional well-being?

I know this might sound kind of hokey, or like you're pretending you're the queen in Snow White talking to her magic mirror, but I swear it works. Just try and let yourself write without censoring or judging it. Try doing this for five minutes every day for a week and see what happens.

It's kind of incredible how our deep self can know things that we've been clueless about, at least at a conscious level. It's easy to assume that we know ourselves really well, and maybe in some ways we do. But being truly in touch with yourself and really trusting yourself means that you're always listening, even when Internal You has something to say that you might not want to hear. (What do you *mean* that glass of wine before bed messes up my sleep?!)

As you heal, you have to give yourself space to meet the present you—who you are right here, right now. It is like baby steps when you are first learning to walk, except you are allowing yourself to be vulnerable to how you actually feel, and not try to tuck it away.

Trust me: I spent so long trying to shove myself into that old square hole. And I got so impatient with my inability to just go back to normal. Plus, so many people around me were acting like I should be able to just shake it off and move on. It was like, *You're feeling better, so what's the problem? Get back in the groove!* But I didn't fit in that groove anymore. I'm a triangle, now, damn it! And I had to claim and embrace my triangle self.

The thing is, truly becoming our own best friends and building that unshakable bond exponentially boosts our capacity to heal. That's because it establishes something essential for our recovery: a deep sense of safety. That's what you gain when you're able to come home to yourself.

And when you have that deep foundation to operate from, you feel empowered to do all kinds of things that once felt impossible. That includes throwing out those old masks. I get it—we can get really attached to our masks. Ironically, one of my favorite photos from my childhood is of me and my Papa—my mom's dad—wearing masks. But this is no longer playtime, and these masks aren't fun, and they're not serving us. So it's time to get rid of them!

TAKING OFF THE MASKS

A little while ago, I heard one of the most incredible things ever. It was a stand-up routine from comedian Tig Notaro. Well, that's not exactly right. Because this show? It was anything but routine. It wasn't rehearsed. It was just truth. Raw, honest expression. And it was moving and hilarious, and like nothing else I'd heard before.

The event was simply called "LIVE." In it, Tig steps out in front of the audience and instead of doing her prepared set, she completely abandons it. Instead, she announces, "Hi, hello. I have cancer. How are you?" And she's not joking. At the time, Tig, who had recently experienced a hellacious series of life and health events, including an extremely difficult battle with *C. diff*, had just been diagnosed with breast cancer. And instead of pulling up her bootstraps, putting on her funny mask, and pretending to be fine, she left the mask behind. Instead, she delivered something that's hard to describe. It was touching, it was deeply human, and somehow, it also managed to be gut-bustingly hilarious. It's truly a must-listen.

The reason I wanted to share it here is because it's such an exquisite example of both the tendency we have to wear masks—to put on a pleasing face to make others more comfortable or conform to expectations—and the incredible things that can happen when we leave them off. One of the funniest bits in the show became about Tig checking in on her audience members quickly after delivering the news she had cancer, seeing how *they* were taking it. "Sir?" she asks. "Sir, are *you* okay?" Which suggests the man is having a more difficult time with the diagnosis than even she is. It was a hilarious and incisive send-up of our propensity to put our own needs aside and care for others, which is such a thing. I can't tell you how strong the urge can still be for me at times to reach for my mask.

In the moment, when we're dealing with our own or others' discomfort over a situation, a mask might feel essential. So often it's our default to shift into a role. I remember so many times when I pushed back on something a doctor told me, only to be shot down. Right away I reached for that Good Patient mask and started hard-core fawning. I did it because I felt like I needed that doctor to help me, and I couldn't risk them disengaging. Plus, from being a Pleaser for so long (you, too?), it was massively distressing to feel like I'd upset someone else. So instead of gently and firmly standing my ground, prioritizing my own self-knowledge and well-being, I gave way.

I've done it in medical settings and in personal relationships. When you have a chronic illness, in so many conversations it becomes clear so quickly that you have to take care of the other person's feelings about it. You see that look on their face, or they have the "You're too much" glaze in their eyes, and you realize that instead of them checking on how you're doing, you've got to care for them and their reaction to how you're doing. But I don't do that anymore. (High five, Tig!)

Before we get into how to stop wearing the mask let's look at why we do it in the first place, and *why* we need to stop.

HOW MASKS MAKE US ISOLATED

There are valid reasons we reach for masks. Mask wearing can be a trauma response. When we sense a threat on some level, it can send us automatically reaching for any tools we think could defuse it. That's what happens when my brain-body wants to shift into fawning mode. Yet there are other reasons, too.

Women, especially, are more prone to wear masks because of our biology. Broadly speaking, we are more geared than men to seek social cohesiveness. Some deep part of us wants everyone to get along, and when we feel something disrupting the vibe, we start looking for ways to restore it. In and of itself, that tendency isn't a bad thing—it's good to have peacemakers. The problem is how we're attempting to accomplish that. When we put on a mask we're putting our own needs last, and that's no good. Plus, on a personal level, though we're trying to restore connection, it can actually have the opposite effect.

Remember in the last chapter, how grief therapist Dr. Moffa said that grief can send us into isolation, and that's really bad for our mental health? The same thing happens when we put on a mask. Outwardly, we might restore some sense of balance or comfort, but internally, it actually cuts us off from others and ourselves. That's because the you that's showing up is a false version of you, and that *feels* terrible. Over the long term, it can contribute to challenges with mental and physical health.

Remember back in chapter 1, I described the experience of being at dinner with friends but feeling like I wasn't really part of it? Instead, it was like I was watching from a million miles away, from somewhere deep in The Shadowlands. *That's because I was wearing a mask.* I was trying to pretend that I was good (because society told me I should be, after all) and that I was just another gal out with her pals having a fun time. But that wasn't what I was feeling inside. I did it because society was telling me I should be good and I should be having a good time. And the result was that I felt terrible. Disconnected from my friends, invisible, and unseen.

Wearing a mask is the loneliest feeling I have ever felt in my life. It keeps you hidden and separate. And the longer it goes on, the worse it gets, and the more distant you feel. I learned that at a very young age, early in my journey with my health when I first started having back pain. Quickly I saw that other people couldn't handle me in so much discomfort, so I adjusted to concealing how much pain I was in. It was easier to survive if I didn't have to manage everyone else's feelings on top of everything else I was going through. It was a survival tactic.

In my conversation with Dr. Maté, he shared some profound words of wisdom on this topic. When we were discussing the patient experience and the emotions that can come up—feelings like shame, anger, sadness, and so on—he continued by saying, "and tremendous isolation, because they're so alone with it." He really saw me, and he saw *us*.

It gets back to that sense of having to manage other people's feelings about what's happening. That, to me, is the loneliest place. Dr. Maté elaborated by saying, "If I am wearing a mask, whether you like me or you don't like me, I'm totally isolated. You don't see me. I'm alone behind my mask." He said we first learn to put on a mask in childhood, when our needs were overlooked by others. In the process, we learn to not trust ourselves. He explained, "Somebody who was seen and heard and therefore had trust in themselves would act differently. If you really trusted yourself and you came to me and you said, 'I have such-and-such an experience.' And I said, 'No, you didn't.' If you trusted yourself, what would you say? 'You must be blind,' is what you would say to me."

That lack of self-belief and self-trust that we experience as patients are directly linked to mask wearing. And then, you might start to feel better physically, but mentally and emotionally you're in The Shadowlands. That's when, as Dr. Maté put it, "You're no longer in survival mode, then all the emotions you haven't resolved, haven't processed, will start arising." And that's why we need to shift out of this behavior and learn to operate from a space of honesty and integrity with ourselves. From a space of authenticity. Because here is the thing: You didn't do anything wrong. Nothing. But sometimes, we think we did, which is why we grab for the mask. But you didn't cause it. When you have a chronic illness, there's this tendency to internalize a really damaging idea: *There's something wrong with me*. Here's another one: *I'm not good enough as I am*.

When we think there's something wrong with us, or that who we are is not okay, it makes us reach for a mask. We think we have to contort ourselves because *we're the ones causing the problem*. And the very last thing we want to be in the whole wide world is inconvenient. So we hide our feelings, making ourselves small. We hide behind a mask, pretending things are better than they are.

But chronic illness isn't something you caused, and it's not a reflection that something is wrong with you. Chronic illness is something that *happened to* you. Period. End of story. It's not your fault. And you have no need or reason to hide. You got me?

Taking the mask off is a choice, and it is yours to make. You're owning your own side of it, and instead of taking this automatic action to caretake for others, you're consciously choosing to leave the mask off. I get it: You might be so used to wearing a mask that it's almost hard to notice when you're doing it. It almost becomes part of your persona. So this might take some time and some real practice on your part, but that's okay. It's worth it.

Plus, the reality is that you can't actually control other people's reactions or feelings, and putting on the mask keeps you in loneliness and separation. It keeps you in The Shadowlands. And that is not a healing place.

For me, one of my biggest challenges is when maskless-me makes other people uncomfortable. For forever that felt like the absolute worst thing in the world to me, and that if I left off my mask, they'd reject me. But guess what I finally realized? *It's okay* if other people are uncomfortable. That's on them. I can tell you from the other side that it feels so much better *just being yourself.* And my nightmare of rejection has yet to come true, but now I know that if it did, I'd be alright! I could handle it. And you can handle it, too.

I get it—it's hard at first. So try going maskless and being the real you with people who make you feel safe. Instead of suppressing your actual feelings and catering to the other person, share what you're really thinking and feeling. Say, politely, that you have a different point of view. Ask the questions you want to ask. Go ahead and respectfully push back. Starting with someone safe will help you build confidence. "Actually, I don't think I want pizza for dinner. I'm really craving Thai food." In time, you can work your way up to the bigger challenges. "I have some questions about that medication you're recommending. Can we talk about some other approaches first? Like, are there lifestyle modifications I could make?"

Here are some questions you can ask yourself to help you put down the mask. I recommend you take some time when you feel relaxed and at ease to go through them, but you can also turn to them when you feel that urge to reach for a mask.

1. When do I tend to put on a mask? What types of situations make me feel like I shouldn't or can't be myself?
2. With what people in my life do I find myself wearing masks? Is it some more often than others? What about our interactions or their behavior makes me reach for a mask?
3. How do I feel when I wear a mask? What might it feel like to leave it off, at least with some people, until I build my confidence to go mask-free?
4. What scares me about going maskless?
5. What are some tactics I can invoke to support myself going maskless? Can I bring a friend to the doctor with me? Can I give myself a pep talk before I call my mom? Can I do a daily (or hourly) affirmation, reminding myself how much I love myself—the real me?

At this point, I have lived here for so long, in this space of authenticity and integrity with myself, that if I even try to put the mask back on, I can't do it. It's just too painful. It feels as if my body and spirit reject it, or as if I am abandoning myself, or that I'm sticking a finger in a raw wound. I can't pretzel myself anymore or pretend I'm better than I am for everyone else. *I can't do it!* And here's the thing: I *won't* do it. I finally choose me. Remember from the last chapter how I went to try biomagnetic therapy and the practitioner said something dismissive about chronic illness and trauma, and I spoke up for myself (and all of us!)? I couldn't just smile and laugh and let him off the hook. I couldn't put on that mask again.

Let others own their discomfort. There is nothing for you to resolve. There is the truth of what has happened to you, and it isn't something you should be ashamed of or feel you need to hide. Getting sick isn't a weakness. After all, what's better for you: being honest or continually telling yourself you are *too much* and putting that damn mask back on your face? What is best for your recovery? You decide.

WHAT AUTHENTICITY IS NOT

I want to be clear here that when I'm encouraging you to be honest and aligned with yourself, that's not saying you should just put everyone else on blast. Authenticity is not a license to say whatever you want, whenever you want, to whomever you want. When we live in integrity, that includes having a sense of compassion for others as well as ourselves. We don't want to just become insensitive PEZ dispensers who say whatever we think.

Committing to living mask-free means you might have to develop a whole new set of tools you've never had before. It's not always easy to navigate the space between honesty and sensitivity, and it can take practice. And to be sure, you'll probably have moments where you are definitely doing more work and putting in more care than the person you're sharing that moment with. But remember, it's actually about *you*, not them. It's about being in integrity *with yourself*. I once read that a boundary is a limit you set with others, but it's a promise you keep with yourself. And I think about authenticity the same way.

It's about acting and speaking in a way that reflects who you truly are. While it can seem at times like it's more about having consideration for others—like when you're putting all that care into choosing the right words—it's actually a gift to you, from you.

Because speaking and acting from your deepest self? It's priceless. And it's so powerful for your healing.

In chapter 7, I shared some of what Dr. Maté said about choosing attachment over authenticity. Dropping the mask is about making a shift and choosing authenticity. As Dr. Maté told me, it's about letting go of that old coping mechanism. Thanking it for its service but recognizing that it's not serving you anymore. (Buh bye, fawning! It's been real.) Now, what he said next is SO IMPORTANT to true healing I felt like I needed to give you a moment to prep. You ready?

Dr. Maté said that choosing authenticity is about "recognizing that that adaptive mechanism that did secure your attachments, way back then, now is actually turning against you." In *The Myth of Normal*, he refers to this mechanism as "the stupid friend." It's "the friend that comes along to help you but doesn't get that its services are no longer required . . . From then I recommend that people notice every time they don't trust themselves and to question what's going on. I mean, question it gently. 'Okay, I didn't pay attention to myself. I didn't listen to my gut feelings. What was I afraid of? And am I still that helpless, isolated, vulnerable, resourceless child? Or are other possibilities available to me now?'"

I asked Dr. Maté how we can learn to trust ourselves again and he said this: "I mean, anybody who even asks the question, 'How can I learn to trust myself again?' is already more resourced than they were as a child, because at least they say, 'Oh, who's the one that's aware that I don't trust myself? Where does that awareness come from?' That awareness is the Self. So, it's right there." And all of this healing and awareness, he says, starts with *compassionate inquiry.*

I'm just going to take a second because that was some real gold there, friend. Just asking yourself these questions shows you that you have more resources than you did before!

The other thing I want to mention calls back to something we talked about in a previous chapter—that idea of different people getting to be in different orbits in your solar system. Being your true self doesn't mean you want to go full-tilt vulnerability and radical honesty with everyone. ("How am I doing? I just had a deep guttural cry," or "Well . . . I just peed my pants a little" or "I am crabby AF. That's how I'm doing.") The fact is that not everyone can handle real authenticity, and if you just go sharing all of you with all of the people all of the time, it's bound not to go well with some of them or create a lot of very awkward pauses. It's not about hiding or pretending but being selective about who gets to see the deepest, squishiest parts of you, and who is better kept at a bit of a distance.

Also, I want to acknowledge that as humans, we're often really bad at relating to one another. How often do you ask someone, or have someone ask you, "How're you doing?" or "How's it going?" What a loaded question, right? Yet mostly we just say, "I'm good!" or "Okay!" or my favorite, "I'm fine!" before they hot potato it back. Well, it can be the same when people ask about your health with a "How are you feeling?" Like, is that a *real* question, or is it more conversational? How am I supposed to respond to that? Do I go for it and tell them? Do I hold back? The only thing I can say to that is: You'll have to be the judge. That means that sometimes you'll step in it and reveal more than you normally do, which might be met with a "Oh shit, get me out of here!" look that appears on the other person's face. When that happens, try not to be hard on yourself. Human communication is fraught with missteps, by all of us. The best you can do, is the best you can do. And beyond that, we can all have a little grace and compassion for others, and for ourselves.

Now, this is all well and good, but let's be real. Like I said before, dropping the mask isn't always easy. Some of this is trial and error. But if this feels really hard at first, that's okay. And it's normal. Remember my friend Lori? I was talking to her about mask wearing and she had some really insightful stuff to share about some of her own experiences. She told me: "I think dating lately has been the biggest place where I struggle with the mask. I think coming out of being so ill and having not been able to participate in age-appropriate things for so long, answering normal questions on first and second dates is stressful. I've chosen to lean into it, but answering the question of, 'When was your last relationship?' and having to admit that it was ten years ago, and explaining what happened since that time is a lot for a first or second date. But choosing to stay in it and admitting that, and keeping the mask off, that is the choice."

So good. So powerful! Lots of conjuring of Lori's brave self right there!

And you know what? You might totally flop at the authenticity thing sometimes. You might lose your cool or accidentally grab the mask. And again, *that's okay.* Perfection is a false target. It's all about just doing your best in that moment, and sometimes your best might look like telling someone to fuck off. Kidding! (Mostly.) Your best might look like that quick, awkward subject change. "Hey, are you caught up on watching *Schitt's Creek*?"

Also, I want to say this again because it's really important. It's not about just running around being open and vulnerable with everyone all the time. It's about trying to always be authentic *with yourself.* And that can look different ways in terms of how you communicate with others.

Remember Tig Notaro and her incredible bravery onstage? Her choice to let an entire audience in on her personal struggles was courageous, no doubt. And also, she was thoughtful about whom she opened up to. Meaning, she didn't share her struggle with a crowd of random shoppers at the supermarket. She shared it with a crowd of people who had paid to see her, meaning they were already, at least to some extent, supporters. So while it was risky, she could likely count on some level of positive response. Plus, she was able to lean heavily on one of her strongest personas: Successful Seasoned Comedian. So while she was genuinely open and authentic, she also had that working for her.

Does this sound like a lot of work? I won't lie, it is. At least at first. Then it gets a lot more natural, I promise. The biggest reason that it's worth the work to learn these skills is that they foster connection, with yourself and others. But most important, they help you get back in touch with yourself and create a space where you're free to be you.

In this chapter, we talked about how to get rid of those masks once and for all! Now that you're learning to get those fabulous new comms skills on board, we'll look at how to take a more active role in your overall care. In short, how to become your own health coach.

TEN

HUDDLE UP! BECOMING YOUR OWN HEALTH COACH

As you know by now, I spent many years being a professional patient. But what you don't know is that before my health saga, I was supplementing my acting career with health coaching and teaching Pilates. Then, my health sent me into a chaotic downward spiral.

In the midst of the storm, I would spend hours and hours in the IV room in a functional medicine practitioner's office. My life had shrunk to the size of the doctor's office, as had everyone's around me. I sat there with my headphones on, watching all of these patients give up their entire days and lives to get treatment. Everyone was so stressed, so sick, and so overwhelmed. I would often think: *How on earth are we supposed to DO IT ALL when we feel like we are drowning?* As I started to get better (still misdiagnosed, but kind of meandering in the direction of improvement) an idea was born, and I went to the doc and pitched him on my big vision.

I told him that, as a patient, I saw his office through a different prism than he could. Sitting there, watching other patients struggle, I knew in my gut that this wasn't the only place they felt lost. There on the front lines, I listened to them complain about feeling totally overwhelmed, feeling like nothing was working, without a clear understanding of what medications or supplements they were taking for what. Saying they forgot half of the things the doctor had said, saying that they found it so hard to be the person "managing" everything, and on, and on. As both a patient and a health coach, I knew how hard it was for patients to advocate for themselves. Their plate is already overfull. Add brain fog to that and OOF, it's like your brain feels like a big bowl of scrambled eggs! With no follow-through or support from the doctor's office, they were on their own. And I saw the toll it was taking on them. Plus, lacking clear guidance, in their desperation and willingness to try anything, they would often try *everything*. And that created its own challenges because sometimes they were doing too much. An advocate could help them work through all of the options and focus on only those that made the most sense for them.

I told the doctor he should add a health coaching practice to aid in patient recovery, and he went for it! As the health coach and patient advocate, I would sit in on patients' appointments, take notes, advocate for them, help them recap afterwards, follow through in the time between appointments, and so much more. Later, after the successful launch of *Kicking Sick*, I went out on my own, into private practice.

It wasn't just the patients in that one practice who were struggling, that's generally the way of it these days. Sadly, a lot of it falls on your shoulders, even at progressive and forward-thinking medical practices like the one where I built out my health coaching practice. My wish is that one day, every doctor's office will offer this kind of support for patients, to not only decrease the burden of healing but also offer a more empowering experience when they come out the other side.

But that day isn't here yet, so instead, I'm giving you my crash course on lassoing all the parts of this wild, untamed patient experience. I'm going to take you through the same pieces of health coaching that I address with my clients, only you're going to learn to be your own coach. It's self-health coaching. Let's look at the areas we'll be addressing.

SIX CATEGORIES OF SELF-HEALTH COACHING

When I work with clients, we look at a few key areas of their life that make a huge impact on their health and well-being. There are six big ones:

- **Doctors:** Who are you with and are they workin' for ya? This includes any kind of doctor, from standard Western docs to functional medicine docs. Your main person.
- **Alternative medicine:** I don't love the word "alternative" because it has this vibe that these approaches are kind of fringe or sketch, know what I mean? But the reality is that many of them have been around even longer than Western medicine, and over the past few decades, many of these approaches have gone mainstream. I mean, even the military uses acupuncture, and they've been doing it for decades! I'm an enormous fan of these types of approaches because I think they are some of the most effective for people with chronic illness when it comes to managing symptoms and improving quality of life.
- **Nutrition:** As they say, you are what you eat! I prefer to call this category "nutrition" or "nourishment" instead of "diet"

because it captures the spirit of my approach, which is to focus less on a rigid way of eating and more on the foods (and drinks) that enhance your life.

- **Movement:** Same thing for this care category. Whereas "exercise" can sound so rigid and programmed, and like something you have to do in a sweaty gym, what it really comes down to is moving your body, and doing it in ways that *feel good*, when you can.
- **Sleep, waking, and personal routines:** This might sound straightforward, but here we're not going to look only at sleep but also at an often-overlooked behavior that contributes to high-quality sleep, and lots of other good stuff. I'm talking about REST, along with overall stress reduction.
- **Essential care:** I've given "self-care" the boot. From here on out, it's all about *essential care* and identifying the routines, behaviors, and even mindset that support Y-O-U.

Got it? Here we go!

ASSEMBLING YOUR A-TEAM

When you have a chronic condition, it often feels like you are free-falling out of a plane with no parachute. You need to put together your A-team, as I like to call it: your A+ list of doctors and other care providers who meet your own personal criteria for a good and solid match for your health care needs.

I encourage my clients to keep their A-team small if they can. You want to keep a "less is more" mentality. Quality over quantity. The more streamlined and intimate your team, the better. So try to focus on a small group of providers who are best equipped to care for you and meet your specific needs.

This core team is your parachute. And it all starts with the right doc.

Top Docs

Both of the first areas of care—doctors and alternative medical providers—have some overlap in terms of how you want to approach them, but we'll first start with more traditional providers.

We've already talked a lot about the medical system. Here we're going to look at ways you can make the most of your medical experience, given the givens. Put on your thinking-smart caps, and let's get to work.

How to Know If Your Doc Is Right for You

Chances are, you're currently seeing one or more medical providers. The big question I explore with my clients, and that I encourage you to ask yourself, is: Are you really being *cared* for?

How do you assess whether you're getting care or just treatment? Here's a checklist of questions to ask yourself:

- Does my health care provider take the time to listen to me?
- Are my interactions with my doctor warm and professional?
- Does my doctor make me feel at ease when I come into the room? Do they make me feel safe and like they can help me?
- Have they seen cases like mine before and have they been successful in treating it?
- Does my doctor have insightful and new ideas for the medical approach?
- Does my doctor communicate with the other people I am seeing and think collaboratively?
- Do I feel like I am making headway between appointments?

- If I have questions about a recommended therapy or course of action, does the doctor consider my questions and concerns and address them respectfully and thoughtfully? Do they want my input?
- Is my current doctor open to discussing approaches or therapies I've researched or heard about?
- When an approach doesn't work, are they thoughtful and collaborative?
- When you come back for a follow-up, have they looked into solutions for you in the interim?
- Does my doctor think about me between appointments and come prepared with thoughts or insights to the follow-up?

The truth is, we are all different and so are our needs. You might have more or different requirements than the ones I've listed here, and that is okay! Take what you like from this list, and toss the rest.

If you consider this list and come up with more NOs than YESes, if you feel like it's up to you to come up with new ideas and steer the ship, like the doctor is doing an experiment with you in unchartered water, or if you feel like you're not making real progress, it's time to move on. No more treading water here, folks! Go and interview new people and make sure they check all of your boxes. Your A-team is out there, and they are yours to find.

Finding the Right Docs

Okay, here is the deal straight up: Choosing the right doctors is as important as any major decision you will make in your life and it should be treated as such. I mean, we want out of this hell hole right?

I get it: Finding the right doc can be hard. In some cases, you might be limited in the type and assortment of docs you have access to. But don't worry, in a minute I'll share some tips and tricks for trying to make the most of your relationship with any health care provider, whether they're a dream doc, or more like a *bad dream* doc. So, we're going to look at how to do the best you can with what you got.

That said, if you're going doc shopping, here are some places to look.

- **Patient recommendations:** One of the best ways to find caring docs who are great at treating your particular illness(eseses) is through recommendations from other patients in the area. You might know some people who fall into this category, or you might have to go hunting. Many chronic illness organizations and social media platforms have dedicated patient groups where you can drop in and ask for recommendations.
- **Searches and lists:** There's the good old Google search, the "best doc" rankings lists, and so on. Any of these can help turn up some options.
- **Doctor recs:** If you know any doctors personally, ask them who they'd send their family to. Good doctors tend to know good doctors. And if they don't know them personally, they often know of the name because they have a good reputation in the doc circles. The same is true with nurses—they often know who the best docs are. Get in with the *in* crowd and ask around!

Here's the deal: *You* are seeking medical care for something that is ailing *you*, so you are in charge. You have the ability to find someone, then either stay with them or fire them as you see fit. Sometimes this comes with a little trial and error, not unlike dating or taking out a new car for a test drive. You probably have to actually do some doc dating—making appointments and talking to them in person—to see if they're a potential match. But the steps above can hopefully help you narrow down the list and weed out the ones who aren't worth your time and energy.

When you meet that new doc, you'll want to ask yourself essentially those same questions as we discussed. Do they listen to you? Do they truly consider what you're saying? And so on. Or better yet, don't just follow my advice and my questions, take a few moments to reflect on what's most important *to you.* After all, these are *your* care providers, which makes you the best (and only) judge of what you need and who is best for you.

Now, I want to talk about someone I see as an essential player on the team of anyone with a chronic illness. A quarterback, if you will.

Functional Medicine Docs

In my opinion, functional and integrative doctors are the best of both worlds because the care they provide is truly wholistic. Functional medicine docs span the space between regular docs (GPs, specialists, etc.) and alternative care providers. A functional medicine doc can be like a one-stop shop, and *I think everyone with a chronic illness should have a functional medicine doc on their team.*

The big difference between regular docs and FM docs is that they have training in areas that regular docs generally don't have, such as nutrition. The upshot is that a functional doc has more arrows in their quiver. They might recommend supplements or dietary changes over meds, though they can prescribe meds, too. They also take a close look at your lifestyle to understand how you're living, how that could be impacting your health, and what changes could help you.

After seeing many, *many* standard doctors, I saw a functional medicine doctor. On the first visit he took a piece of paper and drew all of the systems in the body, including what each does. Then he explained how my symptoms showed that some of the systems weren't working properly. What we needed to do, he explained, was to get every system working optimally and working together. Yes, please!

In my experience, a functional medicine doc is the best core for your team.

BEING A GREAT PATIENT

You want a great doctor, but you also want to be a great patient. To be super clear, this is not about being that Good Patient who distorts yourself in order to not upset your doc. (We don't fawn anymore, my people.) A great patient is a patient who is doing their part to ensure that they get good care. Because in the words of every relationship counselor ever: It takes two! So, in addition to coming correct by prepping for your appointment, here are some things you can do that will help you unlock the Great Patient badge and get the excellent care you need (and deserve!).

How to Talk to Your Doc

When you're working with a new doc, especially, you want to set some ground rules. I like to have a level-up conversation where I tell them how many doctors I have seen and that, as they can see in my medical records, this is not my first rodeo. I explain that what I'm really looking for is a partner to help me get better, and that I really need them to be honest and tell me if there's a point when they think they can no longer help me. Being straight up is the way to go.

You Best Come Prepared

Another tactic to make the most of your time with your doc is to be prepared. Now, getting ready for a doctor's appointment isn't just about taking a shower, brushing your hair, and donning your finest athleisure-wear. It's about putting in some advance thought and making a plan. Here's what I advise my clients:

- **Health history:** My tried-and-true approach is to write down your entire history, in detail, in advance, and try to make it as concise as possible. Then put it down. Come back to it after a day and make sure you are not repeating yourself or missing any important details. The more detail the better, but try not to repeat yourself. For instance, being tired, fatigued, and lethargic are the same thing, so keep it concise. Then, you want to do the same process for your current day symptoms: write it down, step away, make sure it's concise and specific. Bring both this and the health history to the appointment and have a copy you can leave with the doctor for their files.
- **Questions and research:** Come prepared with any questions or research you've found that you'd like to share with your doc.
- **Medical records:** Have any medical records you want to share with the doc? Send them over a week in advance. It takes some time to process this stuff, and it's best if they have your records in hand at your appointment.

What it all boils down to is this little ditty: If you want good care, step it up and be prepared.

Take Notes

You'll want to be sure to take notes at the appointment and to keep a care record. Combined, these help you track what can be a complex process. (*What was the name of that medication I tried last year and what was the dosage?*) All of these things seem so memorable at the time, but as time marches on it can be easy to forget.

I talk to my clients about *memorializing* what happened at the doctor's appointment so you have a game plan between appointments and you're clear on next steps. Again, when you're sitting there with the doc right in front of you, it can be easy to think you'll remember it all. But later you're all, "Wait, am I supposed to take this new medication with food or between meals? And was I supposed to get another blood test now, or wait until my next appointment?" Sure, you could email and wait for a follow-up, but we don't have any more time to waste.

How you take notes is totally up to you. A notes app on your phone, a good old-fashioned pen and a dedicated notebook, voice memos to yourself. Whatever works! Just do it. If you think I am kidding, I literally write notes like I am interviewing Michelle Obama and don't want to miss a single syllable. Trust me: After the very first time you can't remember what the doc said about a prescription or what they want you to tell your other specialist, then you realize you can just look back at your handy dandy notes, you'll thank yourself. After you make your own notes, take a day, then go back and fill anything in that you may have missed.

If possible, I advise my clients to go to their appointments with an advocate, whether it's a health coach or simply someone who loves you. This is someone who can take notes for you and make sure you get your questions answered, so you can be present in the moment. You'll need to give your advocate your list of questions so they can back you up. And if you can't get an advocate to accompany you, everything above stands!

As the appointment is ending, take a minute and scan yourself and all the information you just heard. Make sure all of your questions have been answered and consider whether you have any follow-up questions.

Also, make sure you ask before you leave how to get in touch with the doctor in between appointments should you have any follow-up questions that you think of later.

After the appointment, I ask the doctor's office for a copy of the doctor's notes to make sure I'm not missing anything. That also ensures that I have it to share with other doctors on my team and *not waste time.*

Knowing When to Say "No"

Now, what if you encounter a situation where you disagree with your doc? Like, what if they recommend a course of treatment you're not down for, or if they don't want to try a course of treatment you're interested in? What if you know a med is making you sick and they're dissing and dismissing what you're saying?

Here are some additional red flags to look out for:

- They only recommend one course of treatment or approach without being willing to explore any others.
- They use absolute language, like "This always works," or "That never works," or "This is the only drug for that."
- If you ask why you would be having a negative response to a medication and they just say "I don't know." End of conversation, nothing further to be explored.

As we discussed in the last chapter, the time to stop giving away your power is *right now.* There's a new sheriff in town, and they don't do masks and people pleasing. Remember this: You have a right to say NO to care that doesn't sit right with you. You don't have to stay with someone who isn't truly helping you. This is your one precious life and if someone makes you feel uneasy, it's time to move on. You also have a right to say all kinds of other things Good Patients don't say and to practice authenticity. Here are some examples:

- "I'm not sure—I need time to think about it."
- "I hear what you're saying, but I know my body and that doesn't sound right for me."
- "I'll consider that, but what are some other options or approaches?"
- "Are there any treatments/medications/procedures you know about that I can look into?"
- "If I was your spouse/parent/best friend/child, what would you advise?"
- "If I was going to opt for a non-drug/non-surgical approach, what would you recommend?"
- "What lifestyle factors should I be looking at that could influence my symptoms or outcome?"

Granted, with that last question some will be trained in this and some won't. So know your audience ahead of time. Which brings us to the great world of *alternative* care providers.

ALTERNATIVE CARE PROVIDERS

For our purposes in this chapter, I want to introduce two ideas. The first is that if you're hitting brick walls with "standard" care, I really encourage you to try other modalities, including so-called *alternative* medicine. There are SO MANY out there, and many of them fill the gaps left by traditional care. For instance, modalities such as traditional Chinese medicine and acupuncture (which are often practiced in tandem) address the whole self—not just the whole body, but whole person.

An advantage of these modalities is that most of them don't just look at symptoms. Instead, like functional medicine docs, they look at systems *and how they interact.* They also look at lifestyle factors like your stress level, what you're eating, how you move your body (or don't), and so on.

Sometimes these approaches can be viewed as more on the woo side of things. I want to be clear that I'm using *woo* in the good, insider way. I know some of this stuff might sound a little cray, at least at first, but it can be really effective for patients like you and me. And here's the deal: The truth is we have tried everything and will try ANYTHING to get better.

The main thing is that you need to listen to yourself. It's about tuning in to the modalities that feel safe and good and effective for you. So even if your bestie or your favorite influencer swears by ayurveda, homeopathy, or qi gong, that doesn't mean it's right for *you.* And the reverse can also be true. Even if your spouse looks at you like there's a live frog sitting on your head when you tell them you plan to try sound bathing to help regulate your nervous system, ain't no shame!

The second takeaway that I want to make sure you get is that all those things we just said about medical providers? Well they apply to ALL providers. You deserve *care,* not just *treatment.* If the massage therapist you go to is dialed out or speaks to you disrespectfully, move on! This is *your body* and *your whole self,* and it should be treated with respect by all who approach it.

So that's the general 4-1-1 for care providers, but what about the care you provide yourself? Because when it comes down to it, doctors and other practitioners can do only so much. In the day-to-day and the minute-to-minute, you're the one who has more of an impact on your health and well-being than anyone else. So now, let's shift gears, from the folks who help you, to all the many,

MANY ways you can help yourself! Because let me be clear: No matter where you are in your health journey, there is *always* something YOU can do to help yourself feel better. To improve your circumstances. And to boost your outcomes. Even if it's just a teeny tiny baby step, there is a step you can take. But it's yours to take.

Remember my friend Kira, who struggles with rheumatoid arthritis? She told me that the best, most impactful changes she's made have been to shift some aspects of her diet, start weight training, and add Chinese acupuncture to her regimen. But no one told her to do that. From ages sixteen to thirty-nine, she had to find those solutions on her own! There is a special, individual cocktail that works for each of us, and it's largely up to *us* to find the recipe. Doctors and other care providers can help, but we've got to be the engine driving that train.

There's a difference between treatment—which is what your providers help you with—and symptom management, which is about feeling better. When it comes to what helps you feel better, you're the best and only real judge of that. You with me?

I get it: There are limiting factors. Finances. Time. Energy. And on, and on. Those are all very real. But even within these constraints, I promise you there are still options. And small changes and little routines that make a big difference. I've experienced it myself and seen it with my clients, and I know the same is true for you. And sometimes, just a single visit with a different care provider can make a massive impact! Most of the critical elements for good health—I'm talking movement, sleep, sunlight, breathwork, and community—are all free.

Remember what Dr. Hyman said, that our chosen behavior is the biggest influence on how we feel. Recently, I saw a doctor and she told me something similar. She said: "Doctors tell our patients what to do, but all of the hard work is on the patient to do themselves."

That's the truth. We can turn to docs for help but then it's on us to follow through and do all the hard work. In addition to that very real fact, it's on us to search for additional therapies and modalities that could help us. And when it comes to our lifestyle, it's up to us to get informed, then make healthy choices. No one can do that for us. That is incredibly empowering! Just take it one step at a time, and as you start to feel better, you'll start to feel more motivated to make positive choices and take positive actions because they will start to help you. We can only be as healthy as our environment—externally and internally. This means the air we breathe in our home, the food we eat, the water we drink, the products we use, all the way to making sure our home is as nontoxic as possible. These are key factors in feeling good and living well. And guess what? All of this is up to you to help your body rock.

Okay, so let's explore some of those other lifestyle factors that can impact how we feel in the day-to-day and help us become our own health coaches. We'll get rolling with nutrition.

FORGET THE DIET—FOCUS ON HOW YOU FEEL

Most of us understand that food plays some kind of role in our health and how we feel. But here's the reality: Nutrition is *the foundation* for how you feel. Think of food as your primary lifestyle medicine. It's that important. And it's a way that, on your own, you can help yourself start to feel better. In some cases, dramatically better. Starting in my teens I suffered for years with debilitating back pain—years I spent on anti-inflammatory medication that didn't really help me. Then I switched to an anti-inflammatory diet a decade later, and the pain disappeared! Food really can make that big of an impact on your health. And get this: you can do all of these other things—exercise, get acupuncture, get good sleep, and so on—but if you're not paying attention to what you eat, you're undermining all of it. And I mean *all of it.* "You are what you eat" isn't just a saying, it's a fact.

When you're struggling in one or more areas of your life, it's easy to go to food for a "treat" or for momentary comfort. But while that rush of sugar or saturated fat or salt might feel good in the moment, in the end it's likely to make you feel even worse. Don't get me wrong—I love food. When I was a kid I'd polish off a box of chocolate chip cookies without even thinking twice about it. I was never taught that what you eat dictates how you *feel.* But as part of my healing, I found that eliminating certain foods and food groups made me feel so much better that I started to re-evaluate everything I ate. Then, during the pandemic I fell in love with cooking, and now what I consider a treat is usually something extremely healthy for me, and also extremely delicious.

I've done a lot of research, some of it for clients and much of it for myself. And one thing I've learned is that diets don't work. That's because we think of them as *diets.* As these structured, rigid ways of eating that often involve a lot of denial and deprivation, followed by a binge because it isn't sustainable. Instead of focusing entirely on specific foods that you cut out and what you *don't* eat, I've found it more helpful to focus on what makes me feel good, and what makes me feel good is what *nourishes* me.

Food and *nourishment* are not the same thing. Yes, we need to have some awareness of macronutrients (protein-carbs-fats) and micronutrients (vitamins, minerals, and so on). But I've found that, big picture, if you're paying attention to what nourishes you, these things largely take care of themselves. For instance, I might eat a giant, gooey pizza that might feel good in some way in the moment, but ten minutes later? Not so much. That's because it's not nourishment, but something that lights up my taste buds and my brain momentarily, and then lets me down hard.

Nourishment, on the other hand, makes me feel good—in the moment and throughout the day. It helps me sleep better. It gives me energy. AND it tastes good. So as you consider what your daily intake will include, I've found a helpful question to ask is: "Am I just eating, or am I nourishing myself?" You might know that answer in advance, and it might involve some trial and error of eating things and *really noticing* how they make you feel. Finding the right foods for you can be a practice that unfolds over time. And the right foods might shift over time, depending on where you are in your life, or your cycle, because we are ever evolving. But coming back to this idea of nourishment, and checking in with yourself, is like the rudder on your boat, helping you navigate your nutrition throughout different stages and phases of your life.

I will say that at first, changing your eating habits can be hard. That's why I generally advise my clients to go slow, shifting just one or two things at a time. The good news is that the changes that occur in your body can happen remarkably quickly. Within just weeks (or even faster) your health and even your palate will start to shift. Healthy food will taste like a flavor explosion, and your body will send you signals saying, "More of that, please!"

When making a change, the most important thing to remember is thinking about what is sustainable for you. You want to make small incremental changes to the way you currently eat to make it more of a lifestyle shift than a diet. The point is to find what works and make it stick.

I will say that most of the healthiest ways of eating point to a few essential concepts. My biggest suggestion is to always look at labels and read the ingredients. If you can't pronounce it, or it has a shelf life longer than yours, you probably don't want to be eating it. If you see an ingredient that you cannot understand what it is or is called something way too broad like "natural flavors," you shouldn't be forcing your body to try to digest it. This goes for fast food and anything else that's ultra-processed. One of the biggest problems with all of these foods is that they tend to increase inflammation in your body. Most of us with chronic conditions already struggle from an overload of inflammation. Numerous studies have shown that an anti-inflammatory diet can be really helpful to people like us.

My general approach with people is to start with an anti-inflammatory way of eating and see how that works. If you think of food as medicine, you want to focus on whole, unprocessed or minimally processed foods to reduce inflammation and increase overall health. My general rule of thumb is also to focus on a mostly plant-based way of eating when possible. It's the basics: a lot of vegetables and fresh fruits, healthy fats like avocado and olive oil, legumes, nuts, seeds, whole grains, and lean sources of clean protein. To me that looks like either vegan proteins, or wild-caught fish and pasture-raised, 100 percent grass-fed animals. But ideally, focus on a plant-centric approach. And take it easy on (or avoid altogether) ultra-processed foods, saturated fats, and any refined or processed sugars as these can all trigger inflammation. I'm on the gluten-free, dairy-free, mostly plant-based eater bandwagon for the same reason. I'm also a huge fan of organic food because of the toxic load that pesticides can create, however access and cost can be limiting factors. The Environmental Working Group publishes two lists—the Dirty Dozen and the Clean Fifteen—that can help direct you to which foods are often best to buy organic if you can and which could be fine in conventional form.

These are concepts we generally know to be among the most reliable when it comes to diet and health. Now, I know some of you keto, paleo, low FODMAP, vegan, or whomever people are sitting there itching to say why your way of eating is best. And that may be true for you! I'm not trying to take that away. What I do want to point out is that just because someone has a new plan of the moment, it doesn't mean it's the best plan for you. Notice a pattern here? This is an opportunity to not just follow wholesale what others are telling you to do, but to tune in to yourself and see what really feels and works best for Y-O-U.

In my experience, I don't think there's one single best way of eating for *everyone*. So, I encourage trial and error based on those basic principles, for starters. Some people like to jump in and try a whole diet, because that's what they've heard from others' works. And I say, have at it. But in your attempt to adhere to those rules, please don't lose touch with your deep self. Along the way, ask yourself if it's truly working for you. Ask how it feels in your body and in your soul. Are all cylinders firing? Is everything in alignment? Are you feeling energized after you eat or like a couch potato?

The takeaway is, food isn't just food. You want to try to find the foods that truly nourish you, in all the ways. And you are the best and only judge of that.

MOVE YO BODY

I know that many people who are reading this will not feel as though they have been able to move as much as they'd like. The point of this section is to encourage you to move as often as you can within your own limits and what's best for you. As with nutrition, there is a *ton* of advice out there about what type of movement is more beneficial. Yoga! Pilates! CrossFit! Mermaiding! I'm not kidding, this is a real thing. People put on mermaid tails and swim. There is no shortage of ways to approach fitness. But as with nutrition, I'm gonna zoom way out and go more conceptual with it.

Instead of exercise, I'm going to encourage you think about ways to move your body that appeal to you. That feel satisfying and nourishing (there's that word again!) and, dare I say, fun! Now, if you're fine going to the gym and clocking your 30 on the treadmill or the elliptical, no problem! That's your jam. Who I'm really talking to are those of you who struggle to "exercise" because it sounds like just that—an exercise. As in, a chore.

If you have a hard time with motivation, this one fact might be the single best concept I can share with you: An analysis of meta-studies (basically this means some scientist did a huge number of huge studies and looked at all the data across them) showed that *exercise is more effective than medication at treating anxiety and depression than medication or psychotherapy.* And it wasn't just one or two kinds of exercise, but basically all the kinds of exercise they looked at. Across the board MOVEMENT IS GOOD FOR YOUR MOOD. The most significant impact came from high-intensity exercise. But I know that it's not necessarily appropriate for everyone, so it's a good idea to check in with your doctor first before you start Ninja Warrior–level training.

The other major thing movement does for us is that it helps to restore a positive relationship with our body. If you're anything like me, struggling with a chronic illness has at times made you feel at odds with your own body. *Why are you doing this to me?!* Or, *Why can't you heal faster?! Move it, will you?!* When we can have positive experiences in our bodies, it doesn't just feel good in the moment, it also contributes to our overall healing. It shows us how strong we can be *in our bodies.* We want to get back on the same team with our beautiful bodies, and feeling good through movement can help.

When I encounter clients who are averse to exercise, my goal is to help them break out of the mental box of what movement has to look like. The goal is to find something that's appealing. Maybe the idea of chugging away on the treadmill (a.k.a., the *dreadmill*) or climbing on a spin bike and being shouted at by a hyped-up, over-caffeinated instructor sounds like the seventh circle of hell. I get it! So, what *does* appeal to you?

Maybe the whole gym thing isn't your scene and you'd rather be outside. Great! I have a friend who got into hiking not because hiking, itself, seemed so appealing, or because she loved cargo pants and big clunky boots, but because she loved the idea of being outdoors and getting to see more of nature. The exercise she gets is actually a by-product. Then there are the folks who play pickleball primarily for the social aspect. Or, if you're like me, I love to jump on a mini-rebounder. It flushes my lymph system and it's fun. There are people who hang out with friends (or make new ones) over a shared activity like walking, kickball, or shooting hoops. Then there's Kira and her new favorite activity: weight lifting. She says it not only helps her physically but also mentally. Pumping that iron makes her feel like a BEAST. And who among us wouldn't benefit from a little more of that in life?

The idea is not to push yourself to exercise, but to find things that pull you. What sounds fun? Or at least motivating? Some people are motivated by a sense of accomplishment. They might sign up for a 10k because they want something to work toward. Others are more moved by the interpersonal aspect, or the opposite—a chance to be alone and focus only on yourself. For loads of busy parents, exercise or movement is a crucial part of their me-time.

If you see exercise as a to-do on a huge, long list, you're less likely to do it, or if you do it, to enjoy it. Now, you don't *have* to enjoy movement, but when you remind yourself it's helping you be strong and sane, it's more likely to keep you motivated. It's no longer just a box to check, it's something to look forward to. Something that adds to your quality of life not just physically but also mentally and emotionally. And doesn't that sound better than just a bunch of squats and lunges?

Granted, not everyone has the gift of mobility, especially when you're in the throes of chronic illness. Fortunately, even a small amount of movement can be beneficial if you bring your full attention to it. Light stretching, gentle movement of the hands, stretching your fingers and rotating your wrists and feet, stretching your toes and rotating your ankles, reaching upward with your arms and lightly leaning side to side to open up your spine—all of these can be helpful.

If your argument is that you don't have time, we'll get to that in just a minute. I argue you could at least get up in the morning and go for a walk if you schedule it in (one of my favorite ways to start the day, mind you). But first, one of the biggest benefits of moving your body is how it can boost your sleep.

CALMING THE F DOWN

Waking slowly, taking breaks throughout the day to tune in to you, and setting yourself up for sleep are essential keys in coming home to yourself after MTB. If you are LIT UP with stress from all you're dealing with, and if your nervous system is going full-tilt, YOU MUST CHILL. Healing only happens when we're in that relaxed, rest-and-digest state in our nervous system.

The value of sleep cannot be underestimated. Fortunately, these days, we have a much better understanding of just how essential sleep is for good health and recovery. It's truly where the deep healing happens! And it's a critical part of the program for people with MTB, as is everything that helps you calm the F down. And sleep is a key part of that.

Unfortunately, if you've got a chronically lit-up nervous system, good sleep can be hard to come by. If you have a hard time with sleep (as I do), I encourage you to do some research and reading on how foods and other substances can help or delay sleep.

(Caffeine: No! Magnesium: Yes!) And since all of that is out there and easily accessible, I won't dive into it in detail here. However, I will share some tips that I think can be overlooked that could help set you up for better sleep.

Create a Routine

When I went to a sleep doc to try to get a handle on my sleep habits, she told me that some of the stuff I was doing was actually totally detrimental to good sleep. The good student in me couldn't believe it. Put simply, I was SHOOK as I thought I was practicing good habits for years. For instance, I thought taking a hot-as-I-can-stand-it Epsom salt bath would be a *good* thing to help me relax before bed. But it turns out that the intense heat was actually stressing my system and sending a message to my brain that it was time to wake up, which is definitely not what you want when you're winding down. And that's what you want: to find the things that help to dial down your nervous system in preparation for sleep. And that does not involve binge watching *The Last of Us*, or *Succession*, or any other programming that winds you up. In fact, the research shows that screen time—whether of the TV, laptop, or phone variety—leading up to bed actually keeps us awake.

Just like with nutrition and movement, what works is going to be somewhat specific to you, but you're going for things that—surprise, surprise—*relax* you. When you locate a few of these things, you can blend them into a secret-sauce nighttime mix designed to prep you for some quality sleep. Here are just a few ideas, but I encourage you to experiment and find your own special recipe.

- Turn off overhead lights and use lamp lights, or dimmers, instead. (Bright light cues your body into wakefulness because it sees blaring lights and thinks, "Sun's up!")

- A soothing music playlist or some ambient sounds like singing bowls, chimes, or whatever you find soothing. (There are loads of these playlists online.)
- A relaxing meditation like yoga nidra, where the focus is on down-regulating the nervous system. (Again, tons of these are available for free online. Or you can dial up your favorite relaxing app.)
- Diaphragmatic breathing is a good thing to try as well. (We'll talk about that in more detail in the next chapter.)
- Reading an actual physical book. Don't try to curl up with the latest productivity report from work or be trying to learn Mandarin. Keep it peaceful and simple.
- Do some journaling or write out a short gratitude list. Try to focus on what happened in your day that was positive or supportive. You're not trying to bypass the negative, but right before bed isn't the best time to process those things as they might have the opposite effect of relaxation.
- An hour before bed, get off all screens. Yes, ALL. The brain can't decipher between screen light and daylight.
- Make sure your room is as dark as humanly possible for sleep.
- Cool things down. Set the thermostat to somewhere between 60 and 69 degrees—whatever feels best to you. The cooler temp will send the message to your body it's time to rest.
- Drink some herbal tea or just some warm water. It's surprising how soothing plain old H_2O can be.

Again, these are just some ideas. The point is really that you create some kind of routine that cues your body that it's time for beddie bye, and start it at least an hour before bedtime, giving yourself time to ease in. Because it's really hard to just plop down on your pillow and expect to suddenly shift to sleep mode.

Prioritize Rest

That brings me to another element of getting good sleep, which is getting good *rest*. And it isn't just rest in the form of taking a nap or even putting your feet up for fifteen minutes. It's about getting in the habit of doing personal check-ins throughout the day, and when you feel like you're dysregulated, grabbing even just a few moments to do something soothing. To take a few breaths, repeat a mantra, whatever works for you to turn that hyper-arousal dial down. I encourage you to do this even when you are not feeling particularly dysregulated—to get in the habit of saying, "Hey, body, how we doin'?" consistently throughout the day. In time, all of this helps to rewire your nervous system and make it easier to re-regulate, so these check-ins—these pauses where we really stop and listen to ourselves—are essential for people with MTB.

Try creating a mini-routine. Set a timer to go off at regular intervals throughout the day—maybe every hour or two. When you hear that ding, if you can, pause and take a deep breath in for three seconds, hold three seconds, out three seconds. Then ask yourself three questions: "How am I doing? What am I feeling? What do I need?"

Another idea is to carve out time in the morning for a gentle, slow wake-up, instead of JUMPING out of bed at the first beep of the alarm clock. You can try setting your alarm just five minutes earlier, so when it goes off, you take those five minutes to do some deep breathing, slowly open your eyes, and maybe do some gentle knees into chest and rocking side to side. We want to be easing into the day, and easing in to sleep. So often, we rush through these jam-packed days and then expect to just drop off at night. Then, we're surprised when we struggle to sleep. After all, we're using so much energy, shouldn't we be able to just go lights out at the appointed time? The problem might be that it's too extreme:

expecting to go from wide awake and totally productive to asleep with no in-between. The problem might be that you're not getting enough rest and that starts with how you wake up.

But wait, aren't sleep and rest synonymous? Not so, my friend. Rest is more like downtime. That space when we're awake, but we're not in go-mode. And it's more effective when it's intentional. We have purposeful rest time when we're just, say, reading a book. Or sipping something hot while watching the birds. Or taking a peaceful stroll. In our culture, we almost disdain rest because it's nonproductive. But rest needs to start being its own reward. We need to start seeing it as an essential piece in our overall well-being puzzle. And that's in large part because we're not light switches. We—and our nervous systems—don't do well trying to just shift from on to off. Instead, we're more like those dimmer switches where we just dial it down a bit.

This is also essential for nervous system re-regulation. When you rest, your nervous system is learning to be awake, but chill, and that might be a space it's not used to. Instead of just highs and lows, we want to develop that ability to be in the in-between spaces as well. That will help to minimize that roller-coaster feeling we can get sometimes, where we're pinging from highs to lows in a millisecond.

One of my favorite ways to chill is to GET FLAT! We tend to assume that if it's daytime and we're awake, we should be upright. But just the act of laying down and maybe doing some deep breaths can help your body shift out of the aroused, sympathetic state and encourage it into the more relaxed parasympathetic state, and that's where healing happens.

Obviously you can't lay down during the staff meeting (even if it's on Zoom), so put a pin in this one and do it when you can, maybe when you get home at night. If you have young kids you're caring for, this can also feel like a major challenge. If you can find a few minutes while they're napping or distracted—even two minutes will do!—go ahead and get flat. Or encourage them to do it with you! Put out a blanket and look up at the clouds, or lay on the floor and notice all the things you never saw before about the light fixture on the ceiling. Or take that time when they're falling asleep to lay down next to them. As with all self-care, sometimes you've got to get creative!

Surprise! Everything we've just covered also falls under the category of *essential care* the fundamental behaviors and mindsets that we can engage to tend to our health and well-being. But there's more!

ELEMENTS OF ESSENTIAL CARE

We just talked about the importance of rest. But there's an important idea I didn't talk about, and it not only applies to rest, but to a lot of what we often consider to be self-care. Often, activities that we characterize as caring for ourselves are actually something else. They're about disconnecting from ourselves. About checking out, or numbing. And those aren't actually healthy.

Think about binge watching an entire season of *Top Chef.* It may feel like a "treat," but what it probably is, is *disconnecting.* You see, with true essential care, we're doing things that *nourish* us (yes, I'm saying it again) and help us be more connected to ourselves. To help restore that mind-body link that may have been broken or damaged by, well, *life.* And especially by long-term illness and interactions with the medical system.

I'm not hating on a good movie, show, or video games, but think about the word *binge.* When we binge anything, we're not focused on connection or even true enjoyment. Think about how you feel afterwards. Probably not refreshed, revived, or rejuvenated.

The thing is, there's nothing wrong with some purposeful distraction now and then. I'm a fan! The key word is *purposeful.* When life feels overwhelming or you just need to shift away from everyday demands for a bit, it's okay to engage in a little distraction. To turn on some guilty pleasure viewing, read a trashy novel, etc. But you want it to be just that: purposeful, and time-limited. It's about finding those things that bring you back into connection and alignment.

Growing up, I used to love to sing and play the piano. But when I got sick, as you know, my acting career fell by the wayside. While I haven't decided to jump back into the acting game, I have done something to reconnect with my former joy. I started taking piano lessons again. It's not part of some grand plan or big goal. I'm just doing it for pure fun and enjoyment. To have something in my life that I just like doing, for me. And it's been amazing. It's rewarding, it stimulates my brain, it makes Danny pick up his guitar and start daydreaming about starting a band. (Sorry to burst your bubble, bro, but *not happening.*)

Think about essential care as things that nourish your *essence.* Plus hobbies and pursuits have another benefit. They help to expand your identity. When we're dealing with serious medical issues, it can feel like your identity shrinks like a shriveled balloon down to just one aspect: patient. When we cultivate other areas of our life, we're blowing it back up again.

Maybe you feel like you don't have time for all of this self-directed care. I know that it's fashionable right now to talk about all the time people devote to their routines. This person meditates for two hours every morning. That person does ninety minutes of yoga each day. This person has a morning routine comprised of meditation AND journaling AND gratitude AND exercise AND red light therapy AND sauna AND . . . Oh, man, it makes me tired just thinking about it. Seriously, how do they have the time? I'm not throwing stones. If you have this kind of time you can dedicate to you, do you! But for most of us, that feels totally unrealistic, and so those #goals feel unattainable. And that just makes us feel worse.

The good news is that when it comes to essential care, it's truly not the quantity, but the quality, that matters. You know, one of the reasons that so much of our "self-care" doesn't feel like it's enough is that we're not *really* doing it. You're not just enjoying nice, soothing Epsom salts soak, you're also on your phone or you've got your laptop over there on the bathroom counter and you're streaming *White Lotus.* (Guilty as charged.) Research actually shows that when we're not fully present with things that are otherwise pleasurable, we enjoy them less. Have you ever gone for a "relaxing" weekend away, only you were so mentally dialed in to work, or to some other aspect of life back home, that when you got home you were just as worn out as when you left? (Hand up for me.)

So, two things here. When you're doing essential care, *do essential care.* Be fully present! The second piece is that when we do that—when we are truly doing what we're doing and it becomes an immersive experience—we don't have to do a lot of it for it to be deeply beneficial.

What are your favorite things to get absorbed in? A workout? Cooking a meal? Having some quality time with your partner? Getting engrossed in a novel? Think about it.

Whatever it is, carve out some time to do it. And if you think you don't have it, I challenge you to find just ten or fifteen minutes in your weekly schedule to do it or an hour a month. Those ten minutes you're scrolling on Instagram during your lunch break? Use that time to immerse yourself in that book you want to read. Rather than watching two episodes of *Top Chef* on Saturday morning, watch one and devote fifteen minutes to doing that crossword puzzle or learning that second language. Whatever it is, find some low-bar, totally doable piece of time, and when that time rolls around, commit to doing that thing FULLY. No interruptions, no distractions. *Get absorbed.* If you can do more than that, great. But the thing to understand—to metabolize way down in there at the cellular level—is that the benefit is not about the amount of time you spend doing essential care, it's about the making the most of that time. Truly tuning in to yourself.

Sometimes with my clients I address the idea of stress separately, but here I'm going to fold it under essential care. That's because so much of what we do for essential care also has massive benefits in terms of stress reduction.

I encourage you to do a stress assessment, where you look at different areas of your life (you can start with work, home, and relationships) and see what's causing you stress. For example, when I asked my client Laura to do this and share her results, this is what she came up with:

Work: having to remind the student teacher to copy plans every day, sending end of day roundup notes to the principal, interacting with children who won't listen when I ask them to do something, grading tests and reports.

Home: cooking dinner while trying to do homework with my three kids, doing the dishes, making and packing lunches, giving the kids baths, calling the plumber to fix the boiler.

Relationships: arguing with my husband about finances, feeling like I don't "hang out" with my husband anymore, worrying about my younger brother's health.

When we looked at this assessment together, we tried to come up with small changes Laura could make that might alleviate even one sixteenth of this stress. For example, she could let the student teacher send the roundup notes to the principal, her husband can give the kids the bath while she makes the lunches or vice versa, and rather than calling her brother every few days about his health, she could dedicate one day a week to checking in.

Granted, it's not always easy to address that stress—kids are gonna kid and bills are gonna bill—but even if you can dial it down just a notch or two, like from an eight to a six, that can be a huge improvement. And hopefully some of the essential care you're engaging in can create some *stress offsets*, balancing out your overall well-being.

It will probably take some practice to figure out what works best to destress you. Is it a drop of essential oils on your palm and three deep breaths? A downward dog and some other stretches? Five minutes outside? Whatever you land on, the trick is to incorporate these little breaks throughout your day as mini-routines. I aim for four times a day, but do what works for you. If you have trouble remembering, try setting a reminder on your phone and practice something for even just two minutes.

Essential care can also include other people and making connections outside of yourself. I'm talking about finding a *community of care*.

FINDING YOUR COMMUNITY

True story: When I was making notes for this chapter, I wrote that it was important to find people you can be *funerable* with. At first I thought it was just a funny typo, but then I realized there is something cool and true about that word, so I'm keeping it!

You do need people you can be funerable with. People who can see the full you: cranky, sensitive, fun-loving, hangry and all! In other words, people who you can be completely and totally yourself with, at all times. We talked about that in the last chapter, on not wearing masks, but I just wanted to mention it again here because it's so important.

There's another dimension of community that I haven't talked about, and that's peeps like you and me. People who know what it is to do battle with the many-headed dragon of chronic illness. A few years ago, a friend popped up and told me they had an extra, last-minute ticket to a fundraising gala for Lyme disease. Did I want to go? Don't mind if I do! I was conjuring beads and sparkles and passed hors d'oeuvres. I didn't picture what else happened.

Sitting there hearing all the speakers talk about their experiences with Lyme disease, so many of which I shared myself, and listening to all the incredible research and the advances in awareness—I was overwhelmed. I was incredibly at ease around thousands of strangers, and it was because they all got it, and they got me. And it was the first time in a long time my mask came off. It was like I'd found my people! A group I never really knew existed. I mean, obviously I knew tons of people have Lyme, but I didn't realize what it would feel like to be with so many of them. To see myself and my life mirrored in so many other people's eyes. It was truly moving. And across the table was a woman who has become one of my dearest friends in the world. I get her, and she gets me.

Fortunately, thanks to the interwebs you don't have to rely on free last-minute gala tickets or in-person meetings to find your people. But I can attest to the value of connecting with this kind of community. To feel so seen, and to know you're not alone—it's powerful in ways words can't really describe. Plus, it has other benefits. Circling back to where we started this chapter, people who have some of your same challenges can be an excellent resource when it comes to everything from doctor recommendations to researching your medical options.

So here we are. This is one of those chapters you'll probably want to revisit a bunch of times as you continue on this journey. But now you have a sense of the basics of self-health coaching, and you can dive in! Grab that steno pad and your favorite pen, and let's keep going.

Next up, we're going to look at some other ways to approach our healing, by engaging help with our mental and emotional health.

ELEVEN

RETRAIN YOUR BRAIN (-BODY)

When you experience MTB, it's the result of a lot of retraining and mis-wiring that's gone on in your brain-body. We've already talked a bit about some of the how and the why that's happened. But now we're getting to the really juicy stuff—the *What you can do about it.* Because that's the good news: Your brain-body can get retrained and rewired. In other words, you don't have to just live with MTB. After all, that is the whole point of this book.

Now, I want to say something big here. It's something I've not only experienced for myself in my own healing, but something that the mental health professionals I interviewed for this book also emphasized. And that's this: When you start to heal trauma, you start to create more space inside yourself by processing and healing these wounds. And something happens. It's like everything inside you that wants to be healed suddenly gets in line. I'm not just talking about your MTB, but *everything.* Even stuff from your childhood—heck, even back to the womb—that your brain-body might not even consciously remember.

Know that this is completely totally normal. And it's actually a really good thing because stuff is showing up that's ready to heal. But also, that's why it's so incredibly important to have people on your care team who know how to help you deal with all of this, over the long haul. And that's what this chapter is all about. As patients, we often normalize situations that are not okay, and then they come up for the taking later, when there's space to deal with them. Think about it: How many times have you been dismissed or invalidated? And how many times have you brushed it off as normal? Once you start to heal from MTB, you begin to realize how not normal and not okay so much of what has happened to you is. This starts with getting sick in the first place. It's tragic. Yet then when we start to heal, what we've pushed down and dealt with bubbles up. The good news is we can finally resolve it and move on!

In the last few chapters, we started to explore some of the basic steps you can take to set your ship right. Or at least to start on that path. I've said it before and I'll say it again: The healing process can be long, and it isn't easy. But it's *totally* worth it.

Healing from any major wound takes time. And often, healing isn't a linear process, meaning some days it can feel like you're really making progress, then others seem more like two steps forward and three step back. That's not an easy road. An irony about healing is that it doesn't always *feel good*. Have you ever had a cut or a scratch and when it starts healing it gets super irritated? (Gives me the willies just thinking about it!) If so, you get me. So, healing requires dedication. Like, to not pick at the scab that's forming no matter how much it itches!

Seriously, though, rather than *dedication*, I actually like to use another word. I think that true, deep healing requires *devotion*. What I love about that word is that it conjures so much more than just dedication. It invokes not just the stick-to-it aspect, but some of the why you're going to stick to it in the first place. Because you're devoted. What are you devoted to? You. Hanging in there with your healing process is a powerful act of self-love.

Now, if you've ever been in a long-term relationship, you know that there are ups and there are downs. You may always love your significant other, but relationships by their very nature just aren't always smooth sailing. But you hang in, and you do the work, and you offer some grace and compassion because you don't just love that person, you're devoted to them. You want things to work. This is the kind of relationship we need to have with ourselves if we want to heal. And I'll tell you something really cool. Maybe you *don't* have that kind of relationship with yourself right now. Maybe there's some resentment. Maybe you've taken you for granted here and there. Well, this process of healing can help to heal that, too. Meaning, it can actually help to repair or simply strengthen your relationship with yourself.

That retraining and rewiring I mentioned a minute ago? The thing to understand is that it's not like rebooting a computer and returning it to factory settings. Remember: There's no normal to go back to. What you're creating is that new normal. And ideally, that new normal is a better normal than the normal you knew before. Including developing a better, closer, more lovey-dovey relationship with yourself. How does that sound?

I hope it sounds amazing because here's the OTHER thing: In order to heal, you gotta really want to heal. No half-assing here, friend. That's not gonna get it done. And that's why devotion is so important. Every time you get impatient and fed up, feeling like things just aren't clicking, that feeling and that commitment is what's gonna keep you coming back to the process. Gently. Lovingly. Taking that deep breath and saying, "Okay, let's keep going." That doesn't mean you can't take breaks. In fact, I encourage it! Say it with me: THIS ISN'T ABOUT PUSHING THROUGH. It's about checking in with yourself, learning what you need, and administering that essential care as needed.

Now that we've covered all of that, let's cut to commercial. This commercial is for something that's helped me out a lot, including helping me get in closer touch with myself and process everything that's happened in my big, long healing journey thus far. What I'm talking about is the practice of *journaling*. I'm a fan. And if it's not already something you do, I encourage you to try it. I'm talking about just an informal, routine practice of recording your feelings. Or, if you're not into journaling, finding some other way to express yourself, even if it's just saying how you feel out loud. I find free writing to be super helpful. That's where you sit down with no particular agenda or structure in mind and just take a little time to write out whatever comes up. It can be really incredible to see what bubbles up from the depths of your subconscious, and again, I've found it to be a great support for me in my healing. In this chapter, we'll discuss a variety of brain-body healing modalities, and I highly recommend journaling as a trusty companion in these processes. It's also a great release. Better out than in, as they say.

That said, grab your snorkel and let's get to diving! We're going to take a look at some of the practices I've found to be especially helpful when it comes to working with MTB. I'm presenting these modalities in no particular order, because what works best for each of us can be different. And it can also change over time. You might make a lot of progress with one approach, but then essentially get to the end of where it can take you, and it's time to switch. Or you might want to add in another modality to give things a boost. It's up to you to decide! Also, there are loads of other approaches out there that I won't cover here—not because they're not potentially amazing, but because I can't cover everything in one book and, more important, I don't have experience with them myself. So I don't feel like I can offer an informed assessment. But I encourage you to do your own research and go ahead and try what feels right and appealing to you. Later in the chapter, I'll offer some general advice on how to figure out if a modality, and provider, might be right for you. But for now, let's take a look at some of the approaches I've benefited from.

TALK THERAPY

For starters, there's good old-fashioned talk therapy, which is generally what we think of when we say "therapy." You sit there with a psychotherapist (a counselor, psychologist, or psychiatrist), either in person or virtually, and, well, talk. These types of therapists also practice different modalities, but there are so many different kinds I'll just encourage you to do your homework. For instance, there's *psychodynamic therapy*, where you explore how your thoughts and past experiences are affecting your current experience of life. There's the *humanistic* approach, which emphasizes personal development and self-awareness. There's *mindfulness-based therapy* which incorporates—you guessed it—mindfulness, to help manage anxiety and stress. The list goes on.

If you're interested in a specific modality, obviously you'll want to find a therapist who practices it. Or, if you're not sure what to try, you can reach out to a few therapists and ask what modality or modalities they practice, and what those involve. Whatever approach you choose, you want to be sure that the therapist is trained in dealing with trauma. This is essential! Bonus points if they have experience dealing with medical trauma and trauma from chronic illness. That almost seems like a no-brainer, right? I mean, what talk therapist wouldn't be trained in trauma? But the fact is that many actually aren't, so you need to ask. In my case, I went to one for years without really getting to the root of the root or the bud of the bud. Just telling me to "take deep breaths" when I was anxious was not going to cut it.

My road took me from talk therapy to CBT, to EMDR, to a somatic approach. As my needs shifted, and as I learned more about what works for me, I added different approaches to my arsenal. And that's been invaluable for my healing, so I encourage the very same for you.

In a minute, we'll go into a little more detail about how to find a therapist who's right for you, regardless of modality. But first, let's touch on just a few of the approaches that could be especially helpful for addressing MTB.

COGNITIVE BEHAVIORAL THERAPY (CBT)

I'm a fan of therapy, period. But for a long time, I equated *therapy* with psychotherapy, and more specifically, with talk therapy. I've done talk therapy for years, well before I realized I had MTB. At that time, I thought therapy was straightforward. You talk, they listen, and maybe they offer some pointers on managing the stuff that's making you feel stressed or anxious. And that can be super helpful. But as I've learned, for someone dealing with chronic health issues, including the invisible wound of trauma, talk alone just wasn't cutting it. After all, there were things going on inside me that I wasn't even aware of. And, as I've discovered, deep, long-term nervous system dysregulation isn't something you can just talk or think your way out of. Though learning to address unhelpful thought patterns is a really helpful tool in your healing toolbox. And that's what I found so helpful about cognitive behavioral therapy, or CBT.

We talked about CBT a little in chapter 7, looking at some basic concepts and practices. Here, I wanted to share a little more, from the standpoint as an overall modality. As I mentioned, one of the things I've found CBT especially helpful for is calming those initial flare-ups, when Super Freak lands on the scene and gets me really amped up in ways that aren't actually helpful.

When I talked to Dr. Peter Levine, the creator of Somatic Experiencing (which we'll talk about in a sec), he said something that was really relevant here. I mentioned to him that when fear comes on me, I feel so afraid, so fast, it feels like a wildfire. He said, "That's a good image. It is like a wildfire that's just burning out of control. Sometimes these are talked about as being *triggers*, but they're more than that. These are explosions of symptoms and chaotic energies, and until we learn to calm those energies, then we're going to be susceptible to those eruptions. And so it takes practice and it takes guidance, but having worked with literally tens of thousands of people and often people with these kinds of physiological symptoms, I know that people can learn to ride those waves and to not become overwhelmed."

That's what I've found CBT (among other modalities) helpful for—riding those waves. When those waves come, CBT is designed in large part to help us *respond* to them rather than just *react*. To calm things down enough that we can relate to what's happening from a more rational and thoughtful place. And we can learn to differentiate between vigilance, which is helpful, and hypervigilance, which is the territory of Super Freak.

I've found that CBT is extremely successful in helping me feel a sense of agency over my thinking. That I don't have to be led by or believe thoughts that are not true, or helpful. Because it engages our brain and our conscious thoughts, CBT is considered a *top-down* approach. Modalities such as somatic experiencing, which are more body-based, are considered *bottom-up*. I like using a mix of both. A kind of meet-in-the-middle approach to cover all the bases. You might decide that you prefer one over the other, and that's totally cool.

In chapter 7, we talked about the SUDS scale and using it to step back and self-evaluate. That's one way of creating distance between you and whatever set your current wave of hyper-arousal a'wave-ing. As CBT practitioner Dr. Lindsay Tulchin told me, "One of the most important things to do is noticing when your fight-or-flight is activated, and then engaging in exercises to activate rest-and-digest and deactivate fight or flight."

A first big go-to for this is to regulate your breathing. One technique is called *diaphragmatic breathing*, and essentially it boils down to belly breathing. It's easiest when done laying on your back, but you can sit on a chair or the floor if necessary:

1. Place one hand on your belly and the other on your chest.
2. Breathe in slowly through your nose and imagine the air is all going into your belly, like you're inflating a balloon. You'll feel the hand on your belly start to rise. If the hand on your chest is rising, adjust.
3. When the "balloon" feels full (but not to bursting), slowly breathe out through your mouth, gently pursing your lips. Envision and feel the balloon shrinking as your belly flattens.
4. Repeat for five minutes, or until you start to feel calm.

Another technique is *box breathing*, which is also simple:

1. Inhale through your nose for four counts.
2. Hold your breath for four counts.
3. Exhale through your mouth for four counts.

4. Hold your breath out for four counts.
5. Repeat anywhere from one to five minutes, until you start to feel calm.

This is how Dr. Tulchin described the impact of these techniques: "Anything where you're really slowing down your respiration rate will then hopefully start to send a signal to your amygdala, which is the part of your brain that is activated. It will send a signal that you're not in danger because you can't do that [kind of slow breathing] if you're running away. And then that hopefully will start to slow down your system enough so that your SUDS will start to go down a bit. And then you can decide, 'What do I want to do now?'"

Another effective, tried-and-true tool I keep in my back pocket is something I think of as *the power of the pause*. As I mentioned in chapter 7, you'll be surprised how much giving yourself an hour or more—even a full sleep—away from something will create the distance you need to see things more rationally. A simple pause can create space for you to evaluate the situation and take some of the intensity out of its sails. Plus, a pause of even just twenty minutes creates enough time for those chemicals of arousal to empty from your system.

Another favorite CBT technique of mine is super simple, at least in concept. In this practice you notice what you're thinking, and label it. For example, when Super Freak flies in from outta nowhere and starts super freaking, I take a deep breath and just listen to her. Often she's saying something along the lines of: "You're going to get sick again, and it's going to be as bad as last time. You won't be able to deal with it, so let's get ahead of it NOW!" Instead of hopping on this thought train with her, observer me steps forward with her clipboard and glasses. Her job is to *listen and label.* "Hmm," she says. "I hear what you're saying. You're feeling scared and anxious." Then I take it a step further and say, "But are these things actually happening right now or are these just my emotions about it?" When I do this, I'm brought to the present moment and can see that I'm actually safe and okay. I'll repeat to myself that I'm alright. I'm just having an emotional thought. What do you think? That sounds doable, right?

What these CBT techniques do is help to calm the initial freak-out down enough that I can remind myself that I can handle it. I can better trust myself. The scary thought of getting sick again is that I won't be able to handle it. But that's not true.

Since I first got sick, I have upped my Lyme game and my life game big-time. I know so much more and I have so many tools. So I know that if something does happen, I'll be able to put on my big-girl pants and deal with it. And I tell myself that: *I can handle whatever happens.*

Again, it's about putting space between you and your reaction, shifting your brain from panic mode into a more intellectual, logic-based mode. That shift dials down the activity in your emotional center. Presto! It's kinda like magic. Notice that what I'm not trying to do is deny or turn off my feelings and my reaction. I'm accepting it. That's important because you don't want to get into a mode where you're suppressing your emotions. You're riding the wave, remember? Not trying to push it back into the ocean.

Before we move on, I want to mention one of my absolute favorite distancing tools, and it's one that I've actually been using this entire book! It's humor. Sure, humor can be an avoidance technique, but it can also be thoughtfully deployed, to lighten things up when they get a bit too heavy or you just need a break or a bit of mental space. In that way, humor is actually a powerful tool to help moderate our reactions to difficult situations or circumstances.

And when we're hit by a wave, one way to create distance and calm our emotions is to have some levity about it. That's why I created Super Freak! Thinking about her always makes me smile, and that makes my hyper-arousal a little less hyper.

There's a lot more to CBT than I've covered here. Basically, you can think of CBT as a set of action-oriented techniques that we can use to help ourselves get clear and move through what we are feeling. It is empowering. But CBT might not be enough for some. On my journey, I found that I was still encountering some blocks, so I got curious about another approach, called EMDR.

EMDR

EMDR stands for eye movement desensitization and reprocessing. That's a mouthful, I know! But it's actually a fairly simple technique, and one that can produce some pretty incredible results. Unlike CBT, EMDR is aimed primarily at treating trauma. It does this by helping people (like me!) process disturbing, stressful, or otherwise upsetting thoughts, feelings, or memories linked to trauma.

I interviewed EMDR practitioner Barry Herbach, and he said that he sees the process as having two pieces. To explain them, he used the example of a car accident. Say his client was driving along and suddenly they get into a crash. While his client ends up being okay, the guy in the car in front of them experienced some pretty horrific injuries and died. The client saw this, and the memory of seeing this man is burned in their brain, causing a lot of ongoing stress and trauma. Herbach said his first goal would be to *desensitize* his client from that mental image. As he put it, "They would no longer be haunted by it, or it have that sting." But there was a second part of the accident. While his client was okay, her son suffered injuries and had to be airlifted to a hospital. She felt tremendous guilt about that. The second aim of EMDR would be to help shift her emotions around the incident so she felt less guilty. To take the charge out of her feelings.

So, how does all of this magic happen? Through directed eye movements. To put it simply, the therapy involves thinking for brief periods of time about a disturbing or heightened incident or memory, while also focusing on an external stimulus. So while you're recalling an upsetting memory, the therapist is holding a pencil that you follow with your eyes in a prescribed series of movements. The external stimulus could also be something like tapping or listening to different sounds.

Okay, so why and how does *that* work? As Herbach explained, "The brain and eyes are interconnected." In fact, technically speaking, the eyes are actually part of the brain. When you were growing in the womb, your eyes basically *formed from your brain.* How wild is that? So, the theory goes that these eye movements link to how the brain functions. Think about it like this: If I asked you to recall a childhood memory, your eyes would move a bit while you're thinking. That's because of that brain-eye link. Well, EMDR works backwards, by using eye movements to connect to your brain—specifically, to change the patterns in how your brain is working.

As Herbach said, a lot of the time, when we are in regular talk therapy, we are speaking about our experiences from our *logical* brain. But when you plug in EMDR, you can shift to the *emotional* brain along with the body (or the brain-body), and that's especially important when dealing with trauma, because it's more about emotion than logic. It's like how we said earlier in the book that trauma is an ongoing response to a trigger that's no longer there. So EMDR can help you defuse the emotions and thoughts linked to that trigger.

Herbach was working with a client who was a Vietnam vet. He'd experienced some pretty horrific things during the war and ever since had a really difficult time sleeping. His logical brain told him a narrative (because that's what logical brains do), which was that he was afraid that while he was asleep, the enemy would sneak in. And that's why he couldn't sleep. Makes sense, right? Well get this: When they brought EMDR into his therapy, his emotional brain told a different story. It said that it didn't actually *want* to feel safe! As it happened, the patient had survived several life-threatening experiences, and after those experiences, he'd felt an incredible rush of euphoria and a different kind of engagement with life. And subconsciously, part of him longed to experience those feelings again. Only now he was home and safe, so that emotional piece of him was actually *wanting* an experience of being unsafe. I know, right! When he'd pursued regular talk therapy and the therapist kept reassuring him that he was safe, it actually made him more depressed. EMDR was the key that unlocked what was really going on inside him.

Another client of Herbach's had experienced a lot of medical trauma during her cancer treatment. Sadly, she had received a terminal diagnosis, but she wanted to undergo chemo to prolong her life. The problem was that, due to her medical trauma, she was terrified. As Herbach explained, "When we've experienced a long-term illness such as cancer, it's extremely difficult for most of us to shift from feeling so unsafe to suddenly feeling like things are okay." It's like our brain-body didn't get the memo. So she got EMDR therapy to help release her fear so she could have the chemo.

One of the things I especially appreciated about talking to Herbach was that he knows all about MTB, because he has experienced it. He had his own terrible dance with Lyme disease, during which he suffered Bell's palsy (a kind of temporary facial paralysis). It was such a traumatic experience for him that for TEN YEARS he'd go in the bathroom and periodically his wife would hear him whistle. When his Bell's palsy started, the first symptom he had was that his ear felt clogged. From then on, any time he experienced the smallest bit of congestion he would start to worry. Was it coming back? If he could whistle, it meant the palsy hadn't returned—*but he felt compelled to keep checking.* When his wife would hear the telltale whistle, she'd shout, "You don't have Bell's palsy!" His point was, even though he understood trauma and knew exactly what was going on inside him, he couldn't just stop the process on his own by appealing to his logical brain. And THAT, my friend, is why it's critical to get help.

There's a lot more that could be said about EMDR (and all of these modalities, really) so if it interests you, I encourage you to do some research to learn more.

SOMATIC EXPERIENCING

Now we've come to one of my favorite modalities—*Somatic Experiencing*, or SE for short. This was the missing piece of everything I was doing before! That's because whereas therapies like CBT and talk therapy are top-down approaches, SE is bottom-up. That's because it's body-based. But rather than explain the theory behind that, I'll let the creator of SE do the talking.

As Dr. Peter Levine describes it, trauma presents itself in the mind, but it starts in the body, so that's where we have to go to heal it. Other modalities that take a more thought-based approach can be great complements to somatic work. But as I've experienced, addressing the mind alone won't heal trauma. You've gotta get into the body and let it talk to you.

When we spoke, Dr. Levine told me that when it comes to trauma, the brain-body connection looks something like this:

> *"Just imagine this: You go outside your apartment and you see somebody falling off their bike and they're injured. The brain is primed to recognize threat and to recognize injury. So it sends a message down to what's known as the vagus nerve down into the guts, and our guts twist. Yuck! Now that nerve is 80 percent sensory. The great majority of that nerve is taking information from our guts and relaying it back up into the brain. And then that gets amplified because remember, the majority of those nerves are sensory. They're taking information from the guts, sending it back up to the brain where it gets amplified. It gets regurgitated. So you have what I call a positive feedback loop with negative consequences. So, one of the things we do in SE is we use different exercises to break that cycle."*

In other words, when we've experienced trauma, the body plays it over and over, creating somatic signs and symptoms. That's how our body is communicating with us.

Reading that, can you feel it in your own body? I sure can! Have you ever had that experience, maybe even with something medically related, where something happens and later, when you go to relax, you start playing the memory on repeat? For me, it's often when someone does something that upset me and I wish I'd handled the situation differently. Right when I'm all snuggled up in bed ready for sleep, BAM! There it is, looping like a greatest hit. And every time that loop loops around again, it's magnified, just like Dr. Levine described. Suddenly my body and brain are lit up like a switchboard.

At this point, Dr. Levine shared an awesome and oh-so-simple exercise to quiet down the brain-body when this happens. This is what he said:

"After you have that kind of event, maybe that night you're laying in bed and your guts are twisting, and then all of a sudden you get an image of the injury that you saw later that day. So I'll give you a very simple exercise that can make you feel more settled, more regulated. But it can bring up difficult sensations as well. But usually they'll move through. So the idea is to take an easy full breath and on the exhalation to make the sound Vooo coming from the belly and letting the breath and the sound all the way out. Then just allowing the breath to come in on its own, filling belly and chest. And then again, let the breath and the sound all the way out until it can't anymore and let the breath come in, filling belly and chest. And as you do this, just notice what you're aware of, sensations, feelings, thoughts, images."

Okay, I'm going to press pause because I know you wanna try that. So go ahead. Reread the instructions and *Vooo* away!

What did you think? It's kind of amazing how just that simple exercise can create a big shift. Now, I'll add that, as Dr. Levine mentioned, sometimes when you do even the most basic exercise, like noticing what you're feeling in your body, it can create uncomfortable feelings in your body. It can make your heart race, you can feel a little shaky, and so on. Or you might start having uncomfortable thoughts. Maybe you hop on the worry train or start having upsetting memories. The trick is to not try to run away from them or to push them down. Instead, you're going to *orient*.

This is how Dr. Levine described it:

"First, be aware of the sensation, because the sensations associated with fear will crest like a wave that comes to the shore and then declines and then goes back into the ocean

of sensations and awareness. So just be able to feel enough of your ground—feel how your feet are literally touching the ground, feel your hands and notice the sensation. If the constriction in the gut gets worse or starts to release, if the heartbeat starts to crest and then diminish. Just notice it. If we can follow the sensations, that takes the fang out of the fear. Then we can notice if any thoughts come up like 'This is never going to end.' When people have something like the thought 'This is never going to end,' they often don't realize it's just a thought. I suggest that they preface that feeling/thought with the following words: 'I have the thought that it's never going to end,' or whatever the thought is. Because it's just a thought. It's nothing more. So to work with the sensation in the body and then also to notice what thought is this for."

So good, right? Notice how you can sort of blend these different modalities? One of my favorite tools when I'm starting to feel that freak-out mode is a simple grounding practice I learned from Dr. Levine. It goes like this:

1. Stand or sit (Dr. Levine advises standing if you're able as it's more effective, but only if it doesn't cause a strain). You can do this with shoes on, but you might prefer just socks or with bare feet so you feel more sensations. It's about whatever's comfortable for you. Now, start by noticing how your feet are contacting the ground—whether the floor, rug, grass, what have you. Notice the connection.
2. Start tracking the sensations in your feet. Is your weight more on one foot than the other, more on the balls of your feet than your heels?

3. Allow your feet to spread out and to widen onto the ground and notice that sensation as well. Here he says he'll sometimes imagine a frog's feet, and how they actually suction to the ground. Is the ground hard, soft? Is the texture rough, smooth?
4. Now, notice your knees. Do they feel locked or braced? Can you shift slightly from one foot to the other? Notice the sensations change as you do this.
5. Now sway gently from one side to the other. This actually has the impact of engaging your *vestibular system*, or the system in your body that maintains balance. And that has the effect of helping you feel more *in balance* with the environment.
6. Bring your attention to your center. Your center of gravity is between your belly button and the lower part of your belly. Become aware of that space inside you as you continue to gently sway.
7. Notice your breath coming into your lower belly as you inhale through your nose. Is it cool? Is it heavy? Now exhale and notice your belly pushing out all of that air.

Any time strong sensations or emotions come up, this gentle protocol can help you feel, quite literally, grounded and centered.

These techniques I've just described are super helpful if you get jacked up—in other words, if your nervous system becomes *hyper-aroused*, where you're feeling all that stress or anxiety. But I also talked to Dr. Levine about something else that can happen with trauma, that we haven't talked about as much in this book. That's *hypo-arousal*, or something called *dissociation*. Instead of the fight or flight states, hypo-arousal is the freeze or collapse space that's more characterized by zoning out or going numb. As Dr. Levine put it, hyper-arousal is about being overwhelmed, whereas hypo-arousal is about collapsing into helplessness. As he explained, so often when we talk about PTSD or CPTSD, we think about the hyper-arousal states, but hypo-arousal—or shutdown—is also a common trauma response.

As I said to Dr. Levine, "I think that's something that's pretty universal with people who've struggled with their health: That, one, they go into overdrive while also feeling totally disconnected from their body. And two, they sometimes feel like they're kind of floating above it because their body isn't a safe space."

He replied: "That's right. And often they literally experience themselves as being out of their bodies and maybe even looking down at their body." That's disassociation. To be clear, many of us experience some combination of hypo- and hyper-arousal symptoms. I experience a Slushie of both with a heavy lean on hyper-arousal. It's usually not all one or the other. Anyway, as Dr. Levine described it, disassociation is a "protective mechanism, so that we're not destroyed by these horrible things that happen to us. And when we disassociate, we *leave holes in the fabric of our body awareness*, and those holes will get filled by physical symptoms. So in helping people work with the dissociation, they're also working with healing the physical symptoms."

Okay, time to hit pause again because that was HUGE. "Holes in the fabric of our body?!" Breathe that one in and out for a minute.

That's one of the reasons I think Somatic Experiencing—or whatever kind of body-based practice you might want to try—is so important. When it comes to physical symptoms, trauma can become like the whole chicken-egg question. Did the chronic illness cause the trauma or did the trauma cause the physical symptoms? After you've developed MTB, who knows? The brain-body is so complex and sensitive and those systems so intertwined. But the good news is that you don't have to tease it all out to be able to heal it. It all starts with simply *noticing what you feel in your body.* Yes, that's all. But especially for people who've experienced dissociation, that can be a big challenge, because as Dr. Levine described it, we've got these holes in our body awareness. So when you start noticing what you're feeling (and doing those things like drinking when you're thirsty and peeing when you have to), you're actually starting to repair those holes!

But as Dr. Levine also explained, when the freeze starts to thaw, some of the awareness and sensation that can come rushing in like a wave can feel scary, or uncomfortable. It can send you into hyper-arousal and overwhelm. And that's when you can practice those awesome exercises we just discussed: the *Vooo* exercise, the orienting, and the grounding. Another simple exercise you can do is to identify a particularly happy, particularly strong memory from your past. If things start to feel overwhelming, you can call up that memory and *really feel it.* All the smiles, all the goodness—let it balance out the fear or the overwhelm.

Now, I just shared some SE practices with you, but as both Dr. Levine and Irene Lyon said, it's really good to have a professionally trained practitioner to work with. Sometimes the overwhelm can get really overwhelming, or the freeze stays really frozen, and you need some extra support and guidance. A skilled professional can help you navigate the murky waters of trauma and provide much-needed emotional support. I get it—we don't all have the moolah or just plain access to an in-person provider. Fortunately, today there are a number of telehealth and other app-based services designed to link people with lower-cost mental health providers. Plus, there are tons of videos online that can help you get started, like at somaticexperiencing.com. Pretty much every modality has one or even a bunch of providers offering free tools and information. Plus there's the library! Many amazing practitioners are also authors, such as Dr. Gabor Maté and Dr. Peter Levine.

Now, before we get into finding a therapist who's right for you, I wanted to touch briefly on one more modality, because it's one that can be helpful.

INTERNAL FAMILY SYSTEMS THERAPY

Internal family systems therapy (IFS) sees each one of us as made up of a collection of wounded or protective inner parts. These parts are led or organized by a core Self. Kind of like a spokesperson. The goal of IFS is to help people access these wounded and protective selves and let them have a voice so they can respond to their wants and needs—to understand and unify these internal relationships so we can experience a sense of unity inside ourselves. We do all this by applying a big dose of compassion.

For example, maybe in therapy you realize that the voice of your fear is really your little Inner Peanut speaking. She needs you to hear her and let her know that you're looking out for her and that she is safe. That you're there to snuggle and care for her, and she never has to worry about being unheard again. If that sounds like I'm speaking from personal experience, you got me. In my own work—during an EMDR session, to be specific—I was taken back to a memory in childhood I'd totally forgotten. There I connected with my Inner Peanut, and it was life changing.

Generally, our different selves are born at times in our life where we were wounded, and that wounding stuck with us in some way. In IFS, when you're triggered, you try to slow down and become present with yourself so you can identify who needs to be heard in that moment.

So if the sound of that appeals to you, I encourage you to check it out by finding a therapist who is trained in this approach.

These are just a few of the many, many modalities that can help you work with MTB, and again, I encourage you to do your own research and make your own decisions about what to try for yourself. But I will say that one guideline seems to work really well whatever the approach: Slow and steady! I encourage you to be gentle. That means, be wary of any approaches that feel too intense or require you to *push through* areas where you feel resistance. In my humble opinion, the best way to approach any kind of trauma is not with a wrecking ball, but with kindness, patience, self-love, and self-compassion. (And if you have trouble engaging any of those, we're going to unpack some practices to help with that in the next chapter.)

And remember, if you start down a path and it doesn't feel right, *you can stop*! Take a breather or stop completely and shift to another modality. As Dr. Levine mentioned, you can experience a lot of discomfort in the healing process, but what you don't want to feel is flat-out distress. And again, you don't want to feel like you're supposed to go for the gold medal in trauma healing by pushing. Make sure you're with a therapist and practicing a modality that feels *supportive*, even if the work feels challenging at times.

CHOOSING A THERAPIST

When it comes to choosing a therapist, what do you look for? For starters, you can refer back to chapter 10. Those same principles of looking for physical health providers apply when looking for professionals to support your mental health. Beyond that, here are a few basics.

Before "hiring" anyone, you'll want to interview them. Schedule a time to have an informal conversation so you can ask them a few questions (like about what modality or modalities they specialize in) and describe what you're looking for out of therapy to see if they feel like a good match. It's not just the specific answers you're listening for, but their overall tone and attitude. Do they seem like a good match for you? If you're going with one of the services where you can access mental health care virtually, you'll have the opportunity to input qualities and qualifications that are important to you in a therapist.

The point is, just like when you're searching for a doctor to help with your physical health, you want to go in with a plan. To ask yourself: *What do I want from a therapist?* For example: *I am not looking to lay horizontal on a sofa and speak to myself during a session. I want the therapist to be all up there and in it with me. I want a therapist who is compassionate, forward-thinking, and who listens and provides insights and feedback. I want a therapist who makes me feel at ease and safe to be my authentic self, warts and all.* It's important to solidify this for yourself first.

I want to mention that even if you have a great relationship with your therapist, needs can change over time. You might come to a natural end where you've done all you can with a therapist and it's time to move on—either to leave therapy or move to another therapist or modality. And that's a normal and natural part of therapy, and of healing! So even if things are going well, it's great to pause periodically and re-assess if things are still working for you. Are you still progressing? Does this approach still feel right and effective for you? Or is it perhaps time to try something new? That doesn't mean you have to leave your therapist either. You could be like me when I decided to keep doing CBT but add EMDR to the mix. When it comes to mixing up your own personal wellness mocktail, you are the best bartender! Only you know what is right for you. And it's okay to change course along the way.

I'm going to round out this chapter where we began: by reminding you that to experience healing, you have to want to heal. You have to be willing to show up for yourself, consistently and with love, because no one else can do the work for you. It's all about self-devotion, my dear friend. And if you're not ready to go all in yet, or you need a break along the way, that's okay! You're not training for the next Olympics. But here's the thing: You've already done this for yourself. You have already been so devoted to your physical healing, so you definitely have it in you. You got yourself here and this far. It's just about shifting the prism and applying your resilience to this part of your healing, which is essential to finding that freedom inside yourself. And healing isn't linear, anyway. We all take different paths. So you can change course, take a breather—whatever you need. Because in the end, what it all comes down to is listening to yourself.

Next up, we're going to look at some additional tools and approaches for helping you get more in tune with your brain-body.

TWELVE

SAFE SPACE

There are so many aspects of MTB that are difficult to deal with, but for me, the hardest was that it made my own body and mind feel like they were not places I wanted to be. They were the source of my suffering, and so the simple act of just sitting with myself often felt excruciating. I would have rather been anywhere else but dwelling within them.

Earlier in the book we talked about how chronic illness and MTB rob you of the ability to feel good inside yourself, because after all, your body and your brain are the source of your distress. That's one of the reasons it can feel so appealing to try to distract ourselves with things outside us—food, TV, Sally being a B, you name it. But of all the truths I've discovered on this journey, here is the capital-T truest: In this life, you are all you have. You come in with you, and you go out with you, and at the end of it, all we are left with is how we are with ourselves. When it comes to life, most things that happen are beyond our control. The only thing we can truly control is how we relate to what happens. How we relate to life. And how we relate to ourselves.

With that in mind, this last chapter is dedicated to some practices to help you roll out the welcome mat for you and make YOU a safe space to be.

ACCEPTANCE

In her book *Radical Acceptance* psychologist and meditation teacher Dr. Tara Brach writes: "We don't have to wait until we are on our deathbed to realize what a waste of our precious lives it is to carry the belief that something is wrong with us." The act of *acceptance* is about allowing things to be exactly as they are. That includes allowing *us* to be exactly as we are.

There's an idea in Buddhism that pain isn't what causes suffering, but our resistance to pain. That's any kind of pain—physical or mental. Instead, if we can accept where we are and what's happening, our suffering will diminish or even disappear. Acceptance is a recognition that in the present moment, things simply are as they are. It's about accepting how impossibly difficult all of this feels to us: the pain, the loss, the unfairness. That doesn't mean we *like* what's happening or that we want it to continue, but we can surrender to it. That's not about giving up. It's about *meeting the moment* and saying, "Okay, this is where I am. This is what's happening." Then, you can choose how to relate and respond.

There's another aspect of acceptance that I think is so important with MTB. When you're in this space, it's really common to feel negative emotions toward yourself and want to reject not only your experiences but *yourself.* That can look like impatience with yourself and self-criticism, even self-loathing. When we feel these things, as painful as they are, they're actually a means of avoiding another kind of pain: the pain of acceptance. Of recognizing that you are where you are, period.

The thing is, there is no use in fighting it. And this might feel terribly sad, or painful, or even excruciating, however, it is ESSENTIAL to full healing. What has happened, has happened. That can be hard to be present with, but at the end of the day, all we can do aside from rewire is to surrender to what has happened and accept it on the deepest level.

I feel extra vulnerable with this, and I feel like you might resonate with me here. This took some deep self-discovery work to unwind, but I always blamed myself for my healing not going faster. I now know I did this so that I wouldn't feel powerless. Being sick was too scary and made me feel too out of control. I was hard on myself, my body, and my mind around my illness because in some way it gave me a sense of control. I thought, *If it's my fault, I can change it.* Blaming myself gave me (and maybe you, too?) the illusion of control at a very heavy emotional price. Now I know that's an illusion, but it took me some time to get here. At the time, turning my pain inward was like a survival tool, but not a healthy one. And the whole time I wasn't consciously aware of how my self-blame was "serving" me. Investigating and being with what's actually going on is one element of acceptance. But how do we do that?

In many ways, this entire book is about learning to practice acceptance, but Tara Brach offers a specific technique that can be particularly helpful—it goes by the acronym RAIN:

1. Recognize what is happening. Name it.
2. Allow the experience to be there, just as it is. No pressure to interact with it, direct it, or otherwise change it.
3. Investigate with interest and care. Get curious. What is this? What am I feeling about it?
4. Nurture with self-compassion. Be patient and kind to yourself.

Let's zoom in on that last one for a moment. One of the most powerful tools for acceptance, and for breaking painful cycles with ourselves after MTB, is self-compassion.

In *The Myth of Normal* Dr. Maté writes: "The compassion of truth recognizes that pain is not the enemy. In fact, pain is inherently compassionate, as it tries to alert us to what is amiss. Healing, in a sense, is about unlearning the notion that we need to protect ourselves from our own pain. In this way, compassion is the gateway to another essential quality: courage." Still, compassion—especially toward ourselves—can be one of the hardest things to feel when we're in that down-and-out, self-critical space.

Most people struggle with some amount of self-criticism or lack of patience with themselves already, but MTB can put it in overdrive. When you're trying to just be with yourself and get your healing on, the inner critic sometimes takes advantage of that brain space as an opportunity to chime in. So, how do you turn down the mic on your critic and exercise some self-love instead?

When we learn to practice self-compassion, it gives us access to a lot of great stuff. We not only feel better being with ourselves but also it can improve our mental and physical health, making us both feel and be more resilient. Research also shows that it can make us more motivated to do things that are good for us, like care for ourselves.

There are a lot of ways to practice self-compassion, but one that resonates with me most and that I think is the simplest, is to treat yourself like you would treat your best friend. For instance, imagine your best pal was struggling with chronic fatigue and they were being self-critical: *What is wrong with me? Why can't I just be like everyone else? Why is my body so jacked?!* If you heard this, the last thing you'd do was agree with them, right? That would make you just about the worst BFF ever. Instead, you'd do things like listen without judgment. You'd reassure them. You'd help them gain perspective. *It sounds like you're having a hard time right now. I hear you, and I'm here for you . . .*

So much of the time, we have a handle on what's good and healthy for others, and yet we struggle to act that way with ourselves. For some reason, we hold ourselves to a different standard, like we're not supposed to have hard days (or years). That we're somehow supposed to be stronger than everyone else. (There's that old *toxic resilience* showing its ugly face again.) But we deserve love and acceptance and support just as much as anyone else.

Dr. Kristin Neff—the queen of self-compassion research—offers this great five-minute self-compassion exercise that I think is really profound. Here's my CliffsNotes version:

1. When you encounter a difficult situation—whether it's circumstances outside yourself or some challenging feelings you're encountering (or a combo)—pause, take a deep breath, and say to yourself: "This is a moment of suffering."
2. Next, say this: "Suffering is a part of life." (You can also come up with your own statement, like, "I'm not alone," or "This will pass," or whatever else feels supportive or comforting to you.)
3. Now put your hands over your heart. Feel the warmth of your own touch where your hands are resting on your chest. Now say, "May I be kind to myself." And say it again and again to your heart's content, as much as it takes until you start to feel some kind of lightening or relaxation. You could also riff with some other self-blessings. Here are some of my go-tos:
    - May I be patient.
    - May I appreciate myself and all the work my body is doing to support me.
    - May I forgive myself.
    - May I accept and love myself as I am.

Self-compassion combined with meditation are two of the most powerful tools to help you start to relate to yourself differently, in ways that are healthier and more self-supportive.

MEDITATION

The idea of meditation first appealed to me because I associated it with being at ease. I saw all of these peaceful-looking people sitting quietly and contentedly with their eyes closed, and I thought, *I want a piece of that!* I so desperately wanted to feel at home within myself, but after all that had happened, I was at a loss for how. So, I tried it.

I walked into my very first class determined to take the leap. I was going to become A MEDITATOR. So I grabbed my cushion and gently settled myself on it, just like everyone else around me was doing. I assumed the position. Then, I proceeded to suffer through one of the most grueling hours I've ever experienced. Almost as soon as I closed my eyes I became uncomfortable and wanted to open them again. Not just uncomfortable, I was in agony. My mind started racing with all of these thoughts, worries, anxieties. Picture Super Freak with a megaphone yelling in my ear: *YOU ARE NOT OKAY! YOU CANNOT RELAX!* It felt like all the stress that I had experienced was coming down all at once like an avalanche.

At one point my eyes squinted open because I just couldn't keep them closed anymore. I looked around and it was like everyone else in there was a meditation rock star all tranquil and blissed out. And then there was me. I had zero chill. With every single cell inside me I wanted so badly just to drop to the floor and army crawl under the slit below the door and out of there. It was horrible. And yet somehow, I got myself to try again. And again. And eventually, over many, many sessions, something happened. I did it. I became A MEDITATOR.

My meditation teacher told me that you can't "get good" at meditating. But what meditating *is* about is this: Making the space inside you a safe and welcome place to be. Now I know any thought, fear, or big feeling I have is safe within this place I call home. That there is nowhere to run and nothing to run from.

Many of the ideas and practices we've already talked about are working toward the grand aim of nervous system regulation. Because when you're dysregulated, it's hard to even feel connected with yourself, let alone peaceful. For me, meditation has been one of the essential practices to help me find that peace. Now, not only do I meditate every day, I even look forward to it. Imagine that! It took time, practice, and patience for me to get here, but I'm so glad I hung in. While I know that not every modality works the same for everyone, I am a huge believer in meditation and it's something I absolutely recommend you try. There are so many different kinds of meditation out there, and I encourage you to try different ones until you find the one, or the mix, that's right for you. It's likely that different approaches will feel better at different times based on what you're going through, and the great part is that you can learn as many as you want.

Among the many styles out there, there are mantra-based meditations, where you repeat a phrase or sound over and over. For example, Transcendental Meditation (TM) and Vedic meditation are both mantra-based.

One of my favorites is loving-kindness meditation (also called Metta), which is especially helpful if you struggle with self-compassion. In this practice, you direct positive thoughts and vibes toward yourself, then others, repeating phrases like:

- May I be healthy.
- May I live with ease.
- May I allow myself to be happy.

Say them out loud or in your head—it's up to you. Also, notice the similarity with some of the phrases from the self-compassion meditation. As loving-kindness expert Sharon Salzberg explains: "We repeat certain phrases because within the phrases there are implications about a different way of paying attention." Instead of criticizing ourselves, "we're going to see, 'What's it like when I wish myself well?'"

Another popular form of meditation is called Zen, mostly known for *zazen*, or seated meditation. Like many other forms of meditation, zazen consists of sitting on a cushion or in whatever comfortable position is best for you. You breathe steadily in and out, while you simply notice whatever thoughts pop up in your mind, or what sensations appear in your body. You don't judge them or hang onto them, you just notice them, then notice whatever appears next. Picture a train pulling into a station to pick up passengers and then leaving for the next station. Your thoughts or sensations are coming and going and you're simply noticing them pull in and out of the station. There's no agenda other than to just be a witness to yourself. You know how when you are with someone and they really LISTEN to you? It feels so good to be deeply seen and profoundly heard. This is time for you to do that for yourself in an intimate way.

It can take some practice because for most of us, our natural inclination is to judge our thoughts and feelings, and to cling to them. To try to follow them or figure them out or even suppress them. *Why am I thinking about my grocery list right now? Why am I singing Taylor Swift in my head? I'm such a bad meditator!* But in time, it gets a lot easier. And the best part is that you can take these skills with you off the cushion and out into life. Like when you're at the doctor's office and you find yourself spiraling. You can remind yourself to just take a few deep breaths, notice the thought, then release it.

I actually find this approach easier than the kind of meditation where you try to clear your mind of all thoughts because, I mean, let's be real: My mind isn't clearing anytime soon. But it can become a more tranquil place. Maybe instead of thinking about my schedule next week or wondering if that pain in my neck is something to worry about, I can shift to noticing my breath as it fills my lungs, trying to focus my breathing down in to my low belly, or listening to the sound of the wind blowing through the trees outside. (Okay, truth: I live in NYC, so those rustling leaves I'm hearing are on an app, but still, same effect.)

Another great form of meditation is walking meditation. If the sitting still part feels challenging, this could be your jam. And you can literally do this anywhere. You simply get outside and start walking. If you can get to a park or somewhere a little quieter, that's even better. But for folks living in major cities, you can still do this. The point of walking meditation is to be present as you're walking. I like to get in touch with my senses. So as I'm walking I'll think to myself, *What do I smell? What do I hear? What do I see?* And really taking a moment to notice it. You can also look down at your feet and watch how each foot touches the ground and feel the sensations in your feet as you move through each step. Simply noticing what's around you can have a surprisingly powerful impact on your nervous system. In fact, nature is one of your best co-regulators.

Remember what my meditation teacher told me: There is no "right way to meditate," meaning you don't get "good" at it. That isn't the point. Even seasoned meditators can struggle to find that Zen space. The point is to bear witness to yourself, rather than try to get an A at the practice of meditating. Still, every once in a while, you may experience a transcendent feeling—something like awe.

People who research the emotion of *awe* (yes, there are such people) say that it's actually one of the most powerful emotions to improve our mental health and transform our perspective on life. And nature is one of the most likely places to experience awe. I mean, think about the last time you looked out at a sweeping vista, watched a hummingbird, or just held a flower in your hand and looked at the incredible colors and details . . .

Awe-some Nature Meditation

If you can't get out in nature, here's a meditation exercise from Dr. Dacher Keltner—the king of awe research—that can help you access the same benefits:

1. Find a place where you can sit comfortably, in a position that feels restful.
2. Take some slow, deep breaths. While you're doing that, notice where you're holding any tension in your body and try to release it.
3. Now, think of a place in nature that is meaningful for you. It could be the backyard of your childhood home. The lake that you went to on that vacation last year. The Grand Canyon, wherever. All that matters is that it's significant to you.
4. Once you've got that place in mind, tune in to your senses. What do you see? What do you hear and smell? How does the air around you feel?
5. Next, notice what you're feeling in your body. What comes up for you? What do you sense *inside you*?
6. Finally, feel the wholeness of this place, and of this space inside you. How can this magical place in nature *live in you*? How can you connect with it more in your everyday life?

Pretty neat, right? I love it.

Another popular form of meditation is guided meditation, where you listen to someone in person, online, or through an app guiding you in what to do. Sharon Salzberg has a beautiful loving-kindness session you can check out. Or you can try yoga nidra—a movement-free practice where you get in a comfy position and the instructor talks you through a sequence of progressive relaxation. One of the great things about this practice is that it encourages deep rest, where even though you're technically still awake, your body is so zoned out that you can experience many of the same healing benefits of sleep. Check!

But meditation isn't the only way to tune in and calm down. Another of my favorites is sound healing.

SOUND HEALING

Science shows that one of the best, easiest ways to tap into the nervous system is through sound. I mean, you already know that, though. Think about some of your favorite sounds: a mountain stream, a purring cat, the breathing of your honey as they lay beside you sleeping. I bet just thinking about that sound conjures a sensation of relaxation washing over you. Now think about your least favorite sounds: a leaf blower, a jackhammer, the percussive sawing noise of your honey as they lay beside you snoring. Now how's your body feeling? Sorry about that. Quick, go back to the purring cat!

Sounds aren't just pleasant or unpleasant, they can actually impact how we feel in the world, and inside ourselves. That's why sound healing can be so effective. And one of the things I love about it is that sound doesn't ask anything of you except to just listen. Meaning, you can just let the sound surround you.

Just like with meditation, there are so many ways to work with sound. You can go to an immersive singing bowl workshop, or clap on the headphones and listen to a free session online. But there are also some less obvious ways to incorporate sound into your healing. For instance, I've always been someone who has a hard time waking up in the morning. That's a nice way of me saying I'm a crab apple. Often when my alarm goes off, I feel so jarred, like a fireman who's got to leap up, slide down a pole, throw on her gear, and GO. Recently, I got an alarm clock that's designed to mimic the slow, brightening light of a sunrise, and with it comes the sound of birdsong. And I'm not kidding: GAME. CHANGER. Crab apple no more.

I also listen to Schumann resonances on the regular, like when I'm going about my everyday routine at home. If you're not familiar, these are a series of sounds linked to the spectrum of the Earth's electromagnetic field. Okay, that probably didn't do much to clear it up. They're essentially the sound of the electromagnetic spectrum that surrounds Earth—the Earth's heartbeat, as they're often called, and you can easily find several versions of it on YouTube. Many believe that the resonances—particularly the frequency of 7.83 Hz—has healing benefits, and that listening to it is kind of like nestling your head against the chest of Mama Earth. How's that for some co-regulation?

The point is, sound is like a direct dial to your nervous system, and you want to pay attention to what's in your ears. If you're feeling like you're all worked up, maybe it's time to turn off the techno and shift to some soothing classical or nature sounds. Or do Dr. Peter Levine's exercise where you do some belly breathing and then make a low *Vooo* sound on your out-breath.

It's kind of amazing what a huge impact sound (and vibration) can have on your brain-body. To me, a short sound bath is like the audio equivalent of sticking my face in a bowl of ice water—it's a quick-fix, nervous system reset. And it's one of my go-tos if I'm feeling less-than-peaceful inside myself.

I encourage you to check out different types of sound healing to find what helps to calm you. Whether its Mama Earth's heartbeat, nature sounds like a peaceful stream or nighttime crickets, singing bowls, monks chanting, or white noise, there are apps out there to help you chill, many of which are free.

TRUE RESILIENCE

What all of this comes down to is what I talked about at the start of the chapter: cultivating the ability to be with yourself. To be *in* yourself. To feel present and safe inside you. And to begin to love and appreciate yourself like you deserve. In all honesty, this could be the hardest part of the healing process, but inside you is where all the real healing happens. So if you want to come out on the other side of that MTB tunnel, you've got to develop a loving relationship with yourself.

Still, it requires enormous courage. It's hard to face your big feelings and to truly welcome them. It's hard to confront the truth of your life and your experiences. It's hard to surrender. It's hard to accept. But the good news is that, as with every other practice I've talked about in this book, the more you do it, the easier it will get, and the more natural it will feel.

And it's truly worth the work. YOU are worth the work. And what you'll find is that it will help you develop true resilience. Not the toxic, press-forward, push-it-down resilience we talked about at the start of the book, but a real sense of "I got this" and "I got me." I'm not overstating it when I say that this work showed me who I am at the very deepest level.

While I was working on this chapter, I remembered another story from my childhood. My family was on vacation at the beach. My mom and little me were out in the ocean. While we were jumping the waves (something I loved to do) they were starting to break really far out. We were already some distance from the shore, but they were getting bigger and bigger and faster and faster. My mom was holding my hand, and as we looked out we saw that these enormous waves were about to break on top of us if we didn't do something quick. As the current started to pull us and the first wave loomed overhead, I felt my mom's fingers slip out of mine. I WAS ALONE. I had no choice but to face the wave by myself. I knew in that moment that the only way out was through. Using my instincts and my pool-practiced mermaid skills, I ducked down into the water as low as I could and let the wave crash over me. Finally, I came up as it dipped, lifting my little Peanut head. Then it happened again, and again. Each time, I sank down under the wave moving with it rather than against it. Finally the surf settled. There I was bobbing along, *and I was okay.* I did it! All by myself. In that moment I seriously felt like Wonder Girl.

In the moments before that wave came, I had no idea how strong I was. And it's the same with riding the waves of MTB. Sometimes you've got to sink down low and let the wave pass. Other times you may have to let a riptide carry you out until things calm down and you can swim again. In either scenario, fighting them makes everything ten times worse, and either way, you *will* learn to ride the waves. You will come out the other side into this bright beautiful sunlight that's waiting for you when you emerge from The Shadowlands.

I know you can do it because *you are so strong.* Stronger than you realize.

CONCLUSION

Wendy Palmer was a seventh-degree black belt in the Japanese martial art of Aikido, and a mindfulness practitioner with more than forty years of practice. Not long before she died, she did a podcast where the interviewer asked her how she stays calm and centered. In response, Palmer shared a story about the founder of Aikido, Morihei Ueshiba.

It was during a training session and Osensei, as he was called, instructed the students to attack him. One after the other they came at him with the best techniques they could muster, and over and over again he fended them off so easefully and skillfully that it looked like he was barely even trying.

Afterwards, when everyone was huffing and puffing and the master was standing there calmly, one of the students asked him, "Osensei, how is it that you always stay centered?"

The teacher laughed. "Oh, I don't stay centered," he said. "But I correct so fast no one can see it."

When I heard this story, I felt like it was the perfect illustration of what life is like in the post-MTB world. And, by post-MTB world, I don't mean the land where all has been healed, but the land where you are in the midst of healing. That land isn't full of flat highways, but ups and downs. As I mentioned earlier in the book, just like physical healing isn't a straight line, neither is mental and emotional healing.

Here's the thing: Along your journey *you will be retriggered.* There are times when you'll be doing great, feeling like you're firing on all burners and the world is your oyster. And then, maybe in the very next moment, you can get retriggered. You'll swear you smell mold, you'll feel that cramping in your belly, you'll start to see those sparkly lights that could signal a migraine, and you'll fall into a full-fear panic. Or you'll tune out and go numb. But here's what will be different: *This time you'll have tools. This time*, you'll know how to refind your center. And as the days, months, and years go on, eventually you'll be an MTB master, doing it so quickly no one can tell that you were triggered in the first place.

In time, being retriggered won't seem like a bad thing, it'll just be a thing. One that you know how to handle. And in that, it's like your whole relationship with the idea of being triggered will shift. When it happens, you'll know that you don't have to be overtaken by it. That you're not helpless and instead have a whole arsenal of techniques you can use to manage it. And that's the real foundation of resilience: flexibility. It's the ability to bounce back. To regain center.

You know, there's a beautifully simple and poetic Japanese proverb that I think applies so perfectly here. And it's this: *Nana korobi, ya oki.* It means: Fall down seven times, get up eight.

Because that's what life is, really. It's a series of falling down and getting up again, in different contexts. It's the human experience at its core. As you learn to navigate MTB and put these tools to use, it's not that you'll never fall again, but that you'll get up quicker. And with less dirt and leaves stuck to your butt. And each time you fall down from a challenge or a trigger, it might seem even harder than the last. But when you get up and you conquer, you realize that you were so much stronger than you thought.

Now, before we part ways, I want to say one more thing: Congratulations! Because you just did something incredibly powerful and courageous. You made it through this entire book. You waded through the science, you sat with the big hard feelings. And you did it *all for you*. And that deserves a celebration.

Please, when you finish reading these words, before you go on to the next thing, I encourage you to stop and sit with that. To put that warm hand over your big, beautiful heart and breathe in that good, powerful self-love.

Really feel it.

You know what that tingling fuzzy sensation is? That's coming home.

Welcome back.

ACKNOWLEDGMENTS

Danny—Thank you for seeing me more clearly than I could see myself when I needed it most. I am so grateful to be witnessed by you. I love and cherish you.

Michele Martin—My amazing literary agent. The smartest creative decision I made was hitching my wagon to yours. You are my teacher, mentor, and fierce advocate. Thank you.

Diana Ventimiglia—Editor extraordinaire! Love at first sight. Thank you so much for getting me and getting it. I wouldn't have wanted to do this with anyone else in the world. Thank you so much for giving me the opportunity. You are dazzling.

Kelly Madrone—Once I saw you, I couldn't unsee you. You are a force, and I am so grateful you said yes to this project. Thank you for everything. You are an amazing partner and teacher. You make me ten times better.

The whole team at Balance—You made my dreams come true giving me the chance to work with you. Thank you forever.

Alice Peck—Thank you for the love, care, and fairy dust you gave the beginning phases of this.

My family—Thank you. I love you.

Dr. Galland—To be a patient in your care after so many years of wrong answers is the greatest gift. You have empowered me in ways I could never describe in words. Without you I would have never had the strength to write this for so many. Thank you for giving me my life back.

Lindsay—Thank you for the storms you have seen me through. Nice to meet you, too.

Dr. Asher—I wish you were here to read this. Thank you for hinting at this idea of trauma before I could even comprehend what you meant. You whispered to me. I get it now. So much of this is for you. I honor you.

NOTES

INTRODUCTION: WHAT'S *WRONG* WITH YOU?

xxvi: **nearly 194 million Americans (that's more than 76 percent of adults!)**: Kathleen B. Watson, Jennifer L. Wiltz, Kunthea Nhim, Rachel B. Kaufmann, Craig W. Thomas, and Kurt J. Greenlund, "Trends in Multiple Chronic Conditions Among US Adults, By Life Stage, Behavioral Risk Factor Surveillance System, 2013–2023," *Preventing Chronic Disease* 22 (April 17, 2025): http://dx.doi.org/10.5888/pcd22.240539.

CHAPTER 1: THE SHADOWLANDS

2: **chronic unpredictable stress**: Xing Fang, Shujun Jiang, Jiangong Wang, Yu Bai, Chung Sub Kim, David Blake, Neal L. Weintraub, Yun Lei, and Xin-Yun Li, "Chronic Unpredictable Stress Induces Depression-Related Behaviors by Suppressing AgRP Neuron Activity," *Molecular Psychiatry* 26 (January 11, 2021): 2299–2315, https://doi.org/10.1038/s41380-020-01004-x.

CHAPTER 2: BUMPING UP AGAINST TRAUMA

16: **that episode of *Friends***: *Friends*, season 8, episode 14, "The One with the Secret Closet," NBC, January 31, 2002.

22: **story about a Japanese soldier**: Mark Memmott, "Japanese Soldier Who Fought On for 29 Years After WWII Dies," NPR, January 17, 2014, https://www.npr.org/sections/thetwo-way/2014/01/17/263350879/japanese-soldier-who-fought-on-for-29-years-after-wwii-dies.

25: **flooded with survival stress**: Assael Romanelli, "Flooding: The State That Ruins Relationships," *Psychology Today*, April 28, 2020, https://www.psychologytoday.com/us/blog/the-other-side-relationships/202004/flooding-the-state-ruins-relationships.

26: **In his book *The Trauma Spectrum***: Robert Scaer, *The Trauma Spectrum: Hidden Wounds and Human Resiliency* (New York: W. W. Norton & Company, 2005), p. 6.

27: **In *The Myth of Normal***: Gabor Maté, *The Myth of Normal: Trauma, Illness, and Healing in a Toxic Culture* (New York: Avery, 2022), p. 16.

CHAPTER 3: THE WILD RIDE OF FEAR LOOPING AND THE THREE *E*S

33: **The Substance Abuse and Mental Health Services Administration (SAMHSA) came up with a model**: "National Strategy for Trauma Informed Care Operating Plan," SAMHSA, accessed August 27, 2025, https://www.samhsa.gov/sites/default/files/trauma-informed-care-operating-plan.pdf; SAMHSA, Trauma-Informed Care in Behavioral Health Services: Treatment Improved Protocol (TIP) Series, No. 57 (Rockville, MD: Substance Abuse and Mental Health Services Administration [US], 2015).

34: **As SAMHSA describes it, "[T]rauma results**: SAMHSA, Trauma-Informed Care in Behavioral Health Services: Treatment Improved Protocol (TIP) Series, No. 57 (Rockville, MD: Substance Abuse and Mental Health Services Administration [US], 2015).

36: **"responding to internal cues of a threat**: Robert Scaer, *The Trauma Spectrum: Hidden Wounds and Human Resiliency* (New York: W. W. Norton & Company, 2005), p. 6.

38: **triggered into a fear loop**: Phil Bradfield, "The Trauma Loop," WinShape Homes, accessed August 27, 2025, https://homes.winshape.org/update/the-trauma-loop/.

38: **Trauma expert Peter Levine explains**: Peter A. Levine with Ann Frederick, *Waking the Tiger: Healing Trauma* (Berkeley, CA: North Atlantic Books, 1997).

38: **There are actually multiple models**: Phil Bradfield, "The Trauma Loop," WinShape Homes, accessed August 27, 2025, https://homes.winshape.org/update/the-trauma-loop/; Namrata Jain, "Are You Stuck in a Trauma Loop? Here's How to Break Free," Mint, October 18, 2025, https://www.livemint.com/mint-lounge/wellness/signs-you-are-stuck-in-a-trauma-loop-and-how-to-break-free-somatic-release-11760725058944.html.

39: **Dr. Bruce Perry, a renowned trauma expert**: Bruce D. Perry and Oprah Winfrey, *What Happened to You? Conversations on Trauma, Resilience, and Healing* (New York: Flatiron Books, 2021), p. 89.

41: **When I spoke to nervous system expert Irene Lyon**: Irene Lyon, interview by Amy Kurtz, June 10, 2025.

43: **As Dr. Scaer writes: "There is nothing**: Robert Scaer, *The Trauma Spectrum*, p. 69.

44: **In 2015, Edmondson published a paper**: Donald Edmondson, "An Enduring Somatic Threat Model of Posttraumatic Stress Disorder Due to Acute Life-Threatening Medical Events," *Social and Personality Psychology Compass* 8, no. 3 (March 5, 2014): 118–134, https://doi.org/10.1111/spc3.12089.

44: **For reference, Dr. Bruce Perry describes PTSD**: Bruce D. Perry and Oprah Winfrey, *What Happened to You*, p. 115.

44: **In Edmondson's view, there are significant**: Edmondson, "An Enduring Somatic Threat Model of Posttraumatic Stress Disorder Due to Acute Life-Threatening Medical Events."

CHAPTER 4: ALL THE EFFING *FS*

50: **He said, "Trauma is not what happened to you**: Gabor Maté, interview by Amy Kurtz, June 1, 2025.

50: **In *The Myth of Normal*, Dr. Maté writes**: Gabor Maté, *The Myth of Normal: Trauma, Illness, and Healing in a Toxic Culture* (New York: Avery, 2022), p. 20.

50: **As Dr. Maté explained when we spoke**: Gabor Maté, interview by Amy Kurtz, June 1, 2025.

51: **"Trauma is not in the brain**: Irene Lyon, interview by Amy Kurtz, June 10, 2025.

52: **As Irene Lyon describes them**: Irene Lyon, "What Is the Fawn Response?" Irene Lyon, accessed August 27, 2025, https://irenelyon.com/2020/03/08/what-is-the-fawn-response/.

53: **Psychotherapist Pete Walker**: Pete Walker, "The 4Fs: A Trauma Typology in Complex PTSD," accessed August 27, 2025, https://pete-walker.com/fourFs_TraumaTypologyComplexPTSD.htm.

60: **Irene Lyon has a useful way**: Irene Lyon, "Functional Freeze Explained (my most popular re-release series)," YouTube, January 8, 2023, https://www.youtube.com/watch?v=-qPCzzn-uQA.

61: **Dr. Galland writes, "Three months later**: Leo Galland, *Power Healing: Use the New Integrated Medicine to Cure Yourself* (New York: Random House, 1997), pp. 37–38.

62: **There's another image Irene Lyon invokes**: Lyon discusses this as part of her SmartBody SmartMind program, accessed 2023, https://smartbodysmartmind.com/program-syllabus/.

63: **you can also feel numb**: "Freezing Could Be a Sign of Trauma—Here's What to Know," Charlie Health, December 12, 2024, https://www.charliehealth.com/post/functional-freeze.

CHAPTER 5: THE WILD, WILD WESTERN MEDICAL SYSTEM

69: **In extreme cases of medical trauma**: Michelle Flaum Hall and Scott E. Hall, *Managing the Psychological Impact of Trauma: A Guide for Mental Health and Health Care Professionals* (New York: Springer, 2016), p. xi.

69: **"My own experience of medical trauma**: Hall, *Managing the Psychological Impact of Trauma*, p. xii.

71: **When I spoke to Dr. Gabor Maté**: Gabor Maté, interview by Amy Kurtz, June 1, 2025.

71: **Researchers took a group**: Wendy Levinson and Debra Roter, "Physicians' Psychosocial Beliefs Correlate with Their Patient Communication Skills," *Journal of General Internal Medicine* 10, no. 7 (July 1995): 375–9, https://doi.org/10.1007/BF02599834.

74: **according to researchers, people with anxiety issues**: Natalie M. Saragosa-Harris, João F. Guassi Moreira, Yael H. Waizman, Anna Sedykin, Jennifer A. Silvers, and Tara S. Peris, "Neural Representations of Ambiguous Affective Stimuli and Resilience to Anxiety in Emerging Adults," *Biological Psychology* 182, no. 108624 (September 2023): https://doi.org/10.1016/j.biopsycho.2023.108624.

75: **In 2024, the *American Journal of Medicine***: Isaac KS Ng, Sarah ZL Tham, Gaurav Deep Singh, Christopher Thong, and Desmond B. Teo, "Medical Gaslighting: A New Colloquialism,"

American Journal of Medicine 137, no. 10 (October 2024): 920–2, https://doi.org/10.1016/j.amjmed.2024.06.022.

76: **Harvard Medical School has an article**: Heidi Godman, "What to Do About Medical Gaslighting: If You Feel Like Your Doctor Is Dismissing Your Health Concerns, You May Be Experiencing Medical Gaslighting," Harvard Health Publishing, April 1, 2024, https://www.health.harvard.edu/staying-Healthy/what-to-do-about-medical-gaslighting.

76: **a study of patients with Ehlers-Danlos syndrome (EDS)**: Colin M.E. Halverson, Heather L. Penwell, and Clair A. Francomano, "Clinician-Associated Traumatization from Difficult Medical Encounters: Results from a Qualitative Interview Study on the Ehlers-Danlos Syndromes," *SSM—Qualitative Research in Health* 3, no. 100237 (June 2023): https://doi.org/10.1016/j.ssmqr.2023.100237.

76: **In one survey, a staggering**: Chloe Castleberry, "Know the Facts: A Deeper Look into Medical Gaslighting," She Knows, December 28, 2022, https://www.sheknows.com/health-and-wellness/videos/2687700/medical-gaslighting-statistics/#:~:text=Chloe's%20Most%20Recent%20Stories&text=According%20to%20the%20October%202022,being%20blamed%20by%20your%20doctor.

77: **Tennis phenom Serena Williams**: Serena Williams, "How Serena Williams Saved Her Own Life: Black women are nearly three times more likely to die after childbirth than white women. Serena Williams was almost one of them. Here, in her own words, she tells her story," *ELLE*, April 5, 2022, https://www.elle.com/life-love/a39586444/how-serena-williams-saved-her-own-life/.

78: **He said, "Invisible to whom?**: Gabor Maté, interview by Amy Kurtz, June 1, 2025.

79: **According to an article shared by the American Association for Physician Leadership**: David Ollier Weber,

"How Many Patients Can a Primary Care Physician Treat?" American Association for Physician Leadership, February 11, 2019, https://www.physicianleaders.org/articles/how-many-patients-can-primary-care-physician-treat.

CHAPTER 6: FROM THE PASSENGER'S SEAT TO THE DRIVER'S SEAT

89: **When I talked to Dr. Gabor Maté**: Gabor Maté, interview by Amy Kurtz, June 1, 2025.

95: **He said that in his entire career**: Leo Galland, interview by Amy Kurtz, February 21, 2024.

97: **Dr. Mark Hyman put it this way**: "Mark Hyman: Struggling with Brain Fog, Weight Gain, and Low Energy? It's Likely Hidden Inflammation! (Do THIS to Reverse It)," interview by Jay Shetty, *On Purpose with Jay Shetty*, August 18, 2025, https://omny.fm/shows/on-purpose-with/mark-hyman-struggling-with-brain-fog-weight-gain-and-low-energy-it-s-likely-hidden-inflammation-do-this-to-reverse-it#description.

CHAPTER 7: RIDING THE WAVE

105: **As Irene Lyon framed it**: Irene Lyon, interview by Amy Kurtz, June 10, 2025.

106: **That's where Dr. Levine got the concept**: PsychAlive, "Dr. Peter Levine on the Somatic Experiencing Approach and the Concept of Titration," YouTube, March 10, 2014, https://www.youtube.com/watch?v=AFUZHz6_0XE&t=419s.

109: **Dr. Lindsay Tulchin, and as she explained**: Lindsay Tulchin, interview by Amy Kurtz, May 30, 2025.

111: **that gap between stimulus and response**: "Quote Origin: Between Stimulus and Response There Is a Space. In That Space Is Our Power to Choose Our

Response," Quote Investigator, February 18, 2018, https://quoteinvestigator.com/2018/02/18/response/.

114: **As Dr. Tulchin explained, it starts**: Lindsay Tulchin, interview by Amy Kurtz, May 30, 2025.

CHAPTER 8: CREATING SPACE FOR HEALING

124: **In this particular episode, the matriarch**: *This Is Us*, season 6, episode 17, "The Train," NBC, May 17, 2022.

132: **As she explains, grief is a natural element**: Gina Moffa, interview by Amy Kurtz, May 22, 2025.

133: **interview Dr. Peter Levine, and he explained**: Peter Levine, interview by Amy Kurtz, June 24, 2025.

134: **In her beautiful book, *I'm Not a Mourning Person***: Kris Carr, *I'm Not a Mourning Person: Braving Loss, Grief, and the Big Messy Emotions That Happen When Life Falls Apart* (New York: Hay House, 2023), p. xv.

135: **But as Dr. Mary-Francis O'Connor**: Berly McCoy, "How Your Brain Copes with Grief, and Why It Takes Time to Heal," NPR, December 20, 2021, https://www.npr.org/sections/health-shots/2021/12/20/1056741090/grief-loss-holiday-brain-healing.

135: **As Dr. Moffa told me: "Grief takes endurance**: Gina Moffa, interview by Amy Kurtz, May 22, 2025.

137: **As Dr. Maté put it when we spoke**: Gabor Maté, interview by Amy Kurtz, June 1, 2025.

138: **As grief counselor Seanna Crosbie writes**: Seanna Crosbie, "Secondary Losses: Coping with the Unseen Impact of Grief," Seanna Crosbie Counseling, accessed September 2, 2025, https://seannacrosbie.com/blog/secondary-losses-coping-with-the-unseen-impact-of-grief.

139: **As Irene Lyon told me, when you**: Irene Lyon, interview by Amy Kurtz, June 10, 2025.

139: **As Dr. Moffa told me: "When you're**: Gina Moffa, interview by Amy Kurtz, May 22, 2025.

140: **Dr. Maté also called out**: Gabor Maté, interview by Amy Kurtz, June 1, 2025.

CHAPTER 9: NO MORE MASKS

150: **This is how Irene Lyon described it**: Irene Lyon, interview by Amy Kurtz, June 10, 2025.

155: **a stand-up routine from comedian Tig Notaro**: Tig Notaro, *Live*, Pig Newton/Secretly Canadian, 2012, album.

158: **In my conversation with Dr. Maté**: Gabor Maté, interview by Amy Kurtz, June 1, 2025.

163: **In *The Myth of Normal*, he refers**: Gabor Maté, *The Myth of Normal: Trauma, Illness, and Healing in a Toxic Culture* (New York: Avery, 2022).

163: **I asked Dr. Maté how we can learn**: Gabor Maté, interview by Amy Kurtz, June 1, 2025.

CHAPTER 10: HUDDLE UP! BECOMING YOUR OWN HEALTH COACH

169: **even the military uses acupuncture**: Nicole Bauke, "Battlefield Acupuncture? Yes, It Exists, and the Military Is Using It to Fight Troops' Pain," *Military Times*, February 10, 2018, https://www.militarytimes.com/news/your-military/2018/02/09/battlefield-acupuncture-yes-it-exists-and-the-military-is-using-it-to-fight-troops-pain/.

181: **Remember what Dr. Hyman said**: "Mark Hyman: Struggling with Brain Fog, Weight Gain, and Low Energy?

It's Likely Hidden Inflammation! (Do THIS to Reverse It)," interview by Jay Shetty, *On Purpose with Jay Shetty*, August 18, 2025, https://omny.fm/shows/on-purpose-with/mark-hyman-struggling-with-brain-fog-weight-gain-and-low-energy-it-s-likely-hidden-inflammation-do-this-to-reverse-it#description.

185: **Numerous studies have shown that an anti-inflammatory diet**: Anna Winkvist, Linnea Bärebring, Inger Gjertsson, Lars Ellegård, and Helen M. Lindqvist, "A Randomized Controlled Cross-Over Trial Investigating the Effect of Anti-Inflammatory Diet on Disease Activity and Quality of Life in Rheumatoid Arthritis: The Anti-inflammatory Diet In Rheumatoid Arthritis (ADIRA) Study Protocol," *Nutrition Journal* 17, no. 44 (April 20, 2018) https://doi.org/10.1186/s12937-018-0354-x; Xiaoping Yu, Haomou Pu, and Margaret Voss, "An Overview of Anti-Inflammatory Diets and Their Promising Effects on Non-Communicable Diseases," *British Journal of Nutrition* 132, no. 7 (October 16, 2024): 898–981, https://doi.org/10.1017/S0007114524001405.

185: **the Dirty Dozen and the Clean Fifteen**: "The Dirty Dozen," Environmental Working Group, accessed October 29, 2025, https://www.ewg.org/foodnews/dirty-dozen.php; "The Clean Fifteen," Environmental Working Group, accessed October 29, 2025, https://www.ewg.org/foodnews/clean-fifteen.php.

187: **An analysis of meta-studies**: Ben Singh, Timothy Olds, Rachel Curtis, Dorothea Dumuid, Rosa Virgara, Amanda Watson, Kimberley Szeto, Edward O'Connor, Ty Ferguson, Emily Eglitis, Aaron Miatke, Catherine E. M. Simpson, and Carol Maher, "Effectiveness of Physical Activity Interventions for Improving Depression, Anxiety and Distress: An Overview of Systematic Reviews," *British Journal of Sports Medicine* 57, no. 18 (February 16, 2023):1203–1209, https://doi.org/10.1136/bjsports-2022-106195.

196: **Research actually shows that when we're not fully present**: Stephen L. Murphy, Floor van Meer, Lotte van Dillen, Henk van Steenbergen, and Wilhelm Hofmann, "Underwhelming Pleasures: Toward a Self-Regulatory Account of Hedonic Compensation and Overconsumption," *Journal of Personality and Social Psychology* 127, no. 2 (May 16, 2024): 312–334, https://doi.org/10.1037/pspa0000389.

CHAPTER 11: RETRAIN YOUR BRAIN (-BODY)

207: **He said, "That's a good image**: Peter Levine, interview by Amy Kurtz, June 24, 2025.

208: **As CBT practitioner Dr. Lindsay Tulchin told me**: Lindsay Tulchin, interview by Amy Kurtz, May 30, 2025.

209: **a pause of even just 20 minutes**: "What Is the Fight, Flight, Freeze, or Fawn Response? In Response to Stress or Danger, Your Brain Responds by Either Defending Itself, Running Away, Stopping, or Reconciling," Cleveland Clinic, July 22, 2024, https://health.clevelandclinic.org/what-happens-to-your-body-during-the-fight-or-flight-response.

211: **I interviewed EMDR practitioner Barry Herbach**: Barry Herbach, interview by Amy Kurtz, July 21, 2025.

214: **As Dr. Peter Levine describes it**: Peter Levine, interview by Amy Kurtz, June 24, 2025.

217: **It goes like this**: "Mindful Discoveries: Peter Levine 'Grounding,'" Sounds True, YouTube, November 10, 2023, https://www.youtube.com/watch?v=PGd8nbidqvc.

218: **As Dr. Levine put it, hyper-arousal**: Peter Levine, interview by Amy Kurtz, June 24, 2025.

CHAPTER 12: SAFE SPACE

226: **psychologist and meditation teacher Dr. Tara Brach writes**: Tara Brach, *Radical Acceptance: Embracing Your Life with the Heart of a Buddha* (New York: Bantam, 2004).

226: **There's an idea in Buddhism that pain**: Shinzen Young, "A Pain-Processing Algorithm," December 7, 2016, https://www.shinzen.org/wp-content/uploads/2016/12/art_painprocessingalg.pdf.

227: **it goes by the acronym RAIN**: Tara Brach, "RAIN: Recognize, Allow, Investigate, Nurture," accessed November 4, 2025, https://www.tarabrach.com/rain/.

228: **In *The Myth of Normal* Dr. Gabor writes**: Maté, *The Myth of Normal*, p. 387.

228: **Research also shows that it can make us more motivated**: Dr. Emma Seppala, "The Scientific Benefits of Self-Compassion," Stanford Medicine, May 8, 2014, https://ccare.stanford.edu/uncategorized/the-scientific-benefits-of-self-compassion-infographic/.

229: **Dr. Kristin Neff—the queen of self-compassion research**: Dr. Kristin Neff, "Self-Compassion Practices," Self-Compassion, accessed September 8, 2025, https://self-compassion.org/self-compassion-practices/#guided-practices.

232: **As loving-kindness expert Sharon Salzberg explains**: Sharon Salzberg, "10-Minute Guided Loving-Kindness Meditation with Sharon Salzberg," Lion's Roar, August 12, 2025, https://www.lionsroar.com/video/10-minute-guided-loving-kindness-meditation-with-sharon-salzberg/.

234: **here's a meditation exercise from Dr. Dacher Keltner**: Dacher Keltner, "Happiness Break: Feeling the Awe of Nature from Anywhere, with Dacher," Greater Good Magazine—The Science of Awe podcast, January 26, 2023, https://greatergood.berkeley.edu/podcasts/item/feeling_the_awe_of_nature_wherever_you_are.

236: **I also listen to Schumann resonances**: Karen Fox, "Schumann Resonance Animation," NASA, January 11, 2012, https://svs.gsfc.nasa.gov/10891/.

CONCLUSION

239: **she did a podcast where the interviewer asked her**: Wendy Palmer, "Dragons and Power Recast: Farewell to a Beloved Sensei—Wendy Palmer," interview by Liz Wiltzen, *Tracking Yes*, December 10, 2022, https://www.trackingyes.com/dragons-and-power-recast-farewell-to-a-beloved-sensei-leadership-embodiment-with-wendy-palmer/; Wendy Palmer, *The Intuitive Body: Discovering the Wisdom of Conscious Embodiment and Aikido, 3e* (Berkeley, CA: Blue Snake Books, 2008).

240: ***Nana korobi, ya oki***: "Nana Karobi, Ya Oki: The Essence of Resilience and Perseverance," WatikOn, accessed October 27, 2025, https://www.watikon.com/nana-korobi-ya-oki-the-essence-of-resilience-and-perseverance.

INDEX

Acceptance, 19–20, 226–30
acting as if (reframing tool), 117
agency. *See* self-advocacy
Aikido, 239
alternative care providers, 169, 179–82
American Association for Physician Leadership, 79–80
American Journal of Medicine, 75–76
anti-inflammatory diet, 185
anxiety
  medical trauma paradox and, 74–75
  normalization of, 1–4. *See also* The Shadowlands
A-team of doctors, 169, 170–75, 179–82, 222–24
authenticity
  choosing attachment over, 89–93, 163
  defined, 162–63
  self-trust and, 159–62
  what it is not, 162–66
autonomic nervous system, 51, 150–52
awe, 233–34

"Back to normal," 34, 54, 153
becoming your personal health coach. *See* self-health coaching
belonging, sense of, 135–36
binging, 194–95
box breathing, 208–9
Brach, Tara, 226, 227
brain-body retraining, 201–24
  about, 201–5
  choosing a therapist, 222–24
  cognitive behavioral therapy, 109–10, 115, 206–11
  EMDR, 211–14
  internal family systems therapy, 221–22
  Somatic Experiencing®, 106–8, 214–21
  talk therapy for, 96, 205–6
breathwork, 191, 208–9
bubble (healing boundaries), 142–45
bubble visualization, 144
Buddhism, 226

Carr, Kris, 134
chronic illnesses, residual trauma caused by. *See* Medical Trauma Brain
cognitive behavioral therapy (CBT), 109–10, 115, 206–11
community support
  grief process and, 135–36, 138–40, 145, 157–58
  for self-health coaching, 198–200
compassion (self), 228–30

compassionate inquiry, 163
complex post-traumatic stress disorder (CPTSD), 46–47
compounded medication, 4–5
connection, grief process and, 135–36, 138–40, 145, 157–58
convalescence, 127–32, 138–42, 145. *See also* space for healing
Crosbie, Seanna, 138

Dairy-free way of eating, 185
desensitization, 211–12
diaphragmatic breathing, 191, 208
diets. *See* nutrition and nourishment
disconnecting, 194–95
dissociation (hypo-arousal), 27–28, 45–46, 56, 218–20
distancing tools, 208–11
disturbance in self-organization (DSO), 46–47
doctors, A-team of, 169, 170–75, 179–82, 222–24. *See also* Western medical system
dog bite example, 35
The Dumps, 56–58

Edmondson, Donald, 44–45
Effects (one of the Three Es), 33–36
effing *Fs*. *See* stress responses
Ehlers-Danlos syndrome (EDS), 76
EMDR (eye movement desensitization and reprocessing), 211–14
emotional defusion, 212–13
"emotional" patients, 17–19
enduring somatic threat (EST), 30, 43–47
environmental sensitivities, xxii
epiphany paradox, 102
essential care
  about, 170
  elements of, 194–98
  rebuilding self-trust and, 151–52
  space for healing and, 129–32, 142–45
EST (enduring somatic threat), 30, 43–47
Event (one of the Three Es), 33–36
exercise. *See* movement
Experience (one of the Three Es), 33–36
eye movement desensitization and reprocessing (EMDR), 211–14

Faith in doctors, 88–93
fawn state, 49–56. *See also* stress responses
fear
  normalization of, 1–4. *See also* The Shadowlands
  state of perpetual fear, 40. *See also* fear looping
fear looping, 31–47
  about, 31–33
  brain-body retraining for, 215–17
  enduring somatic threat, 30, 43–47
  functional freeze state and, 62–64
  phases of, 38–43
  stuck in, 37–38
  survival stress response activation during, 56–58
  Three Es model, 33–36, 44
fight-flight state, 49–56, 105, 110, 111–13, 133–34, 139, 208–9. *See*

also stress responses
fire alarm metaphor, 37, 81
flight-fight state, 49–56, 105, 110, 111–13, 133–34, 139, 208–9. *See also* stress responses
flock state, 49–56. *See also* stress responses
free writing, 153–54, 191, 204
freeze state, 49–56, 105, 133, 139. *See also* dissociation; stress responses
functional freeze state, 41, 58–64
functional/integrative medicine doctors, 87, 95–96, 174–75
"funerable" people, 198–99

Galland, Leo, xiii–xvi, 62, 93–96, 97
gaslighting (medical), 67, 75–77
gluten-free way of eating, 185
golden shadow, 89
"Good Patient" identity, 17–19, 26, 175
gratitude journal, 191
Great Patient tips, 175–79
grief, 12, 28–30, 132–40, 145, 157–58
The *Grieving Brain* (O'Connor), 135
guided meditation, 235

Hall, Michelle, 69
hamster wheel of desperation, 13, 39
healing bubble boundaries, 142–45
health coaching, 167–69. *See also* self-health coaching
health history (written), 176
heart-attack survivors, 44
hemiplegic migraines, 6–7, 42, 91–92, 97
Herbach, Barry, 211–14
holes in the fabric of our body awareness, 219–20
humor, 155–56, 166, 210–11
Hyman, Mark, 97, 181–82
hypervigilance, 36, 37–38, 39, 41–43, 46, 55, 207
hypo-arousal (dissociation), 27–28, 45–46, 56, 218–20
hypothyroidism, 4–5
"hysterical" patients, 17–19

Identity
  as "Good Patient," 17–19, 26, 175
  loss of, 136–37, 138
  as "Sick Person," 11, 20
IFS (internal family systems therapy), 221–22
I'm Not a Mourning Person (Carr), 134
"inconvenient" illnesses, 18–19, 159
inflammation and anti-inflammatory diet, 185
integrative/functional medicine doctors, 87, 95–96, 174–75
internal family systems therapy (IFS), 221–22
invisible illness, 70–73, 78–79
isolation, feelings of, 2, 8, 12–13, 139–40, 157–62

Japanese soldier, stuck in survival mode, 22
journaling, 153–54, 191, 204
Jungian psychology, 89

Keltner, Dacher, 234

Kicking Sick (Kurtz), xix, 18, 122, 168

Labels, 11, 12–13, 209–10
Levine, Peter
on completion of fear loop, 38
on discomfort in healing process, 222
on grief process, 133
on nervous system re-regulation, 106–8
on riding waves of fear, 207
on Somatic Experiencing®, 214–21, 236
listen-and-label practice, 209–10
long COVID, 56–58, 111–12
looping. *See* fear looping
loving-kindness meditation (Metta), 231–32
Lyme disease, late stage
author's community support experience, 199
author's diagnosis and experience with, xix–xxi, xxii–xxiv, 21–22
author's fear looping experience, 42–43
other people's stories, 7–8, 213–14
Western medical system's approach to, 66–67
Lyon, Irene
on fight, flight, and freeze responses, 52
on functional freeze, 41, 60–63
on listening to your body, 150–51
re-regulating the nervous system, 105, 110, 220–21
on space for healing, 139
systematic effect of trauma, 51

Managing the Psychological Impact of Medical Trauma (Hall), 69–70
masks. *See* self-trust, rebuilding of
mast cell activation syndrome (MCAS), xxii, 56–58
Maté, Gabor
on dangers of isolation, 140, 158–59
on mask-wearing and self-trust, 158–59, 163
on process of healing, 137
on reductionism in health care, 27
on self-advocacy, 89–90
on self-compassion, 228
on trauma as a psychic injury, 50–51
on Western medical system, 71, 72–73, 78–79, 81
mechanisms of Medical Trauma Brain, 15–30
about, 15–17
grief acknowledgment, 28–30
resilience trap, 17–20, 23–24, 26, 28
survival stress as trauma, 23–28, 33–36, 38, 57–58
waking up to trauma, 20–23
medical gaslighting, 67, 75–77
medical records, 176
medical system. *See* Western medical system
Medical Trauma Brain (MTB)
about, xxv–xxviii
all the effing *F*s, 49–64. *See also* stress responses
author's self-diagnosis, xxiii–xxv
healing from. *See* tools for healing
insights, 15–30. *See also*

mechanisms of Medical Trauma Brain
medical providers' role in, 65–82. *See also* Western medical system
paradox and ambiguity of, 73–75
from the passenger's seat to the driver's seat, 83–98. *See also* self-advocacy
roots of, 9–14
The Shadowlands, 1–14
wild ride of fear looping, 31–47. *See also* fear looping
meditation, 230–35
meeting-the-moment practice, 226
Metta (loving-kindness meditation), 231–32
migraines, 6–7, 42, 91–92, 97
Moffa, Gina, 132–33, 135–36, 139, 157
movement, 169–70, 186–89
Moving on Doesn't Mean Letting Go (Moffa), 132–33
MTB. *See* Medical Trauma Brain
The Myth of Normal (Maté), 27, 50–51, 90, 163, 228

Nature meditation, 234
Neff, Kristin, 229–30
negative-energy protection visualization, 144
negativity bias, 117–18
nervous system
autonomic nervous system, 51, 150–52
dysregulated nervous system, 24–25, 39–41, 54–55, 75. *See also* Medical Trauma Brain
re-regulating the nervous system, 104–18. *See also* re-regulating the nervous system
responding to stress. *See* stress responses
sleep and rest habits for, 170, 189–94
new normal as better normal, 203
"No" statements, 178–79
Notaro, Tig, 155–56, 165–66
note-taking, b patient, 176–78
numbness (dissociation), 27–28, 45–46, 56, 218–20
nutrition and nourishment, 169–70, 174, 182–86

O'Connor, Mary-Francis, 135
one-hour rule, 116
organic foods, 185
orienting, for re-regulating the nervous system, 110–13

Pain, Buddhism on, 226
Palmer, Wendy, 239
pause, power of, 209
peeing, 149
perpetual fear state. *See* fear looping
Perry, Bruce, 39–41, 44
personal health coach. *See* self-health coaching
plant-based way of eating, 185
post-traumatic growth, 102–3
post-traumatic stress disorder (PTSD), 44–47, 219
post-traumatic stress response. *See* Medical Trauma Brain
Power Healing (Galland), 62
power of the pause, 209

procedural memory, 26–27, 36
psychic wound, of trauma, 50–51
psychotherapy, 96, 205–6
PTSD (post-traumatic stress disorder), 44–47, 219

RA (rheumatoid arthritis), 59–60, 181
Radical Acceptance (Brach), 226
RAIN technique, for acceptance, 227–28
reading, 191
reality check, for re-regulating the nervous system, 113–15
recovery period, 127–32, 140–42. *See also* space for healing
red flags, 178–79
reframing, for re-regulating the nervous system, 115–17
re-regulating the nervous system, 104–18
  with cognitive behavioral therapy, 109–10, 115, 206–11
  grief process and, 132–33
  negativity bias and, 117–18
  overview, 104–6
  rebuilding self-trust and, 148–52
  reprograming the stress response, 108–17
  titration as tool for, 106–8
residual burdens, 50–51
residual trauma, from chronic illnesses. *See* Medical Trauma Brain
resilience, 237–38
resilience trap, 17–20, 23–24, 26, 28
rest, 170, 192–94
retraining brain-body. *See* brain-body retraining
rheumatoid arthritis (RA), 59–60, 181
riding the wave. *See* re-regulating the nervous system
routine, for re-regulating the nervous system, 110–13
rubber-band technique, 112–13

Safe space, 225–38
  about, 225
  acceptance and, 226–30
  meditation and, 230–35
  sound healing, 235–37
  true resilience, 237–38
Salzberg, Sharon, 232, 235
Scaer, Robert, 26, 36, 43
Schumann resonances, 236
secondary losses, 136–38
Self, awareness as, 163
self-advocacy, 83–98. *See also* self-health coaching
  author's experience with, 93–98
  new kind of doc-patient relationship, 93–98
  stepping into role of, 88–93
  Western medicine's doc-patient relationship, 83–88
self-care. *See* essential care
self-compassion, 228–30
self-concept, 46–47
self-health coaching, 167–200. *See also* self-advocacy
  about, 167–69
  A-team for, 169, 170–75, 179–82, 222–24
  author's experience with, 167–68
  categories of self-health coaching, 169–70

community support, 198–200
essential care elements, 194–98. *See also* essential care
Great Patient tips, 175–79
movement, 169–70, 186–89
nutrition, 169–70, 174, 182–86
sleep and rest habits, 170, 189–94
self-talk, for re-regulating the nervous system, 111–12
self-touch, for re-regulating the nervous system, 111–12
self-trust, rebuilding of, 147–66
about, 148–49
authenticity, defined, 162–63
authenticity for, 89–93, 159–62, 163
authenticity–what it is not, 162–66
author's experience of loss of self, 147–48
listening to your body, 149–52
mask-free living, 155–62
re-meeting yourself, 152–55
self-trust erosion, 77–80
sense of belonging, 135–36, 138–40, 145, 157–58
The Shadowlands, 1–14
mask-wearing in, 158, 159, 160
normalization of anxiety and fear, 1–4
personal stories, 6–9, 56–58, 59–60
roots of Medical Brain Trauma, 9–14
spiraling pattern, 4–6, 25
shiva, 134–35
"Sick Person" identity, 11, 20
sleep and rest habits, 170, 189–94
social cohesiveness, mask-wearing for, 157–62
Somatic Experiencing® (SE™), 106–8, 214–21
somatic threat, enduring, 30, 43–47
sound healing, 235–37
space for healing, 119–45
author's need for, 119–26
author's process, 134–35, 136–37
boundaries for the healing bubble, 142–45
convalescence, 127–32, 140–42
grief process, 132–40, 145
life on hiatus while being sick, 119–27
visualizations, 140–42, 144
spiraling pattern, 4–6, 25
stored survival stress, 10–14
stress, normalization of, 1–4. *See also* The Shadowlands
stress assessment, 197–98
stress responses, 49–64
about, 49–51
awareness of, 64
fight, flight, freeze, flock, and fawn, 51–58
functional freeze, 41, 58–64
negativity bias and, 117–18
positive aspects of, 53–54
reprograming for healing, 106–18. *See also* re-regulating the nervous system
social strategies, 53–54
survival stress response, 9–14, 23–28, 33–36, 38, 56–58, 90, 115. *See also* fear looping
"the stupid friend," 163

Subjective Units of Distress Scale (SUDS), 109–10, 112, 208, 209
Substance Abuse and Mental Health Services Administration (SAMHSA), 33–36
surrender, 226–30
survival mode, 1–4, 21–23. *See also* The Shadowlands
survival stress response, 9–14, 23–28, 33–36, 38, 56–58, 90, 115. *See also* fear looping

Talk therapy (psychotherapy), 96, 205–6
therapy. *See* brain-body retraining
thoughts, agency over, 207–8
Three Es (event, experience, effects) model, 33–36, 44
thyroid medicine, 4–5
tick-phobia, 42–43
tiger attack metaphor, 37–38
titration, for nervous system re-regulation, 106–8
tools for healing
  about, 101–4
  becoming your own health coach, 167–200. *See also* self-health coaching
  creating space for healing, 119–45. *See also* space for healing
  nervous system re-regulation, 104–18. *See also* re-regulating the nervous system
  no more masks, 147–66. *See also* self-trust, rebuilding of
  retrain your brain (-body), 201–24. *See also* brain-body retraining
  safe space, 225–38. *See also* safe space
  self-correction speed improvement, 239–41
toughness
  resilience trap, 17–20, 23–24, 26, 28
  true resilience, 237–38
tough stuff, normalization of, 1–4. *See also* The Shadowlands
toxic mold exposure, xxi–xxii
training brain-body. *See* brain-body retraining
trauma
  defined as "unhealed psychological wound," 50–51
  defined as "woundedness," 27
  roots of Medical Trauma Brain, 9–14. *See also* Medical Trauma Brain
The Trauma Spectrum (Scaer), 26
true resilience, 237–38
Tulchin, Lindsay, 109–10, 114, 116, 208–9

Ueshiba, Morihei, 239
unmasking. *See* self-trust, rebuilding of
unrelenting state of fear. *See* fear looping

Vooo exercise, 216–17, 220, 236

Waking the Tiger (Levine), 38
Walker, Pete, 53–54
walking meditation, 233

Western medical system, 65–82
  A-team of doctors, 169, 170–75
  author's experience with, 65–68, 77–79, 81–82
  doc-patient relationship changes, 83–98. *See also* self-advocacy; self-health coaching
  faith in doctors, 88–93
  fractured and fragmented treatment, 70–73
  gaslighting in, 67, 75–77
  healthy anger directed at, 80–82
  medical trauma paradox, 73–75
  mindset in, 68–70
  self-trust erosion and, 77–80
What Happened to You? (Perry and Winfrey), 40
Williams, Serena, 77
Winfrey, Oprah, 40
World War II, 22

Yoga nidra, 191, 235

Zazen, 232–33
Zen, 232–33

ABOUT THE AUTHOR

AMY KURTZ is a patient advocate, health and wellness coach and author. She wrote the trailblazing book *Kicking Sick: Your Go-To Guide for Thriving with Chronic Health Conditions* as a reader's guide to managing debilitating conditions and living fully. A distinct voice in the health space, Amy's work has been heralded by Mark Hyman, Kris Carr, and others. Lena Dunham named *Kicking Sick* one of her "Top 10 desert island books of all time" in *New York Magazine*. Amy has been featured on *Oprah Daily*, *Good Morning America*, *The Boston Globe*, *Fox*, and more. She lives in New York City.

RAISING READERS

Books Build Bright Futures

Thank you for reading this book and for being a reader of books in general. We are so grateful to share being part of a community of readers with you, and we hope you will join us in passing our love of books on to the next generation of readers.

Did you know that reading for enjoyment is the single biggest predictor of a child's future happiness and success?

More than family circumstances, parents' educational background, or income, reading impacts a child's future academic performance, emotional well-being, communication skills, economic security, ambition, and happiness.

Studies show that kids reading for enjoyment in the US is in rapid decline:

- In 2012, 53% of 9-year-olds read almost every day. Just 10 years later, in 2022, the number had fallen to 39%.
- In 2012, 27% of 13-year-olds read for fun daily. By 2023, that number was just 14%.

Together, we can commit to **Raising Readers** and change this trend. How?

- Read to children in your life daily.
- Model reading as a fun activity.
- Reduce screen time.
- Start a family, school, or community book club.
- Visit bookstores and libraries regularly.
- Listen to audiobooks.
- Read the book before you see the movie.
- Encourage your child to read aloud to a pet or stuffed animal.
- Give books as gifts.
- Donate books to families and communities in need.

BOB1217

Books build bright futures, and **Raising Readers** is our shared responsibility.

For more information, visit **JoinRaisingReaders.com**

Sources: National Endowment for the Arts, National Assessment of Educational Progress, WorldBookDay.com, Nielsen BookData's 2023 "Understanding the Children's Book Consumer"